In the Shadow of Angels

INTIMATE STORIES FROM A HOSPICE COUNSELLOR

The author welcomes questions and
comments about the book and can be
contacted at dr.breiddal@gmail.com

SUSAN BREIDDAL, PhD

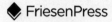 FriesenPress

One Printers Way
Altona, MB R0G 0B0
Canada

www.friesenpress.com

Photos and cover design: Jane Johnston PhD

Mandala photo: Rob D'estrube

I hold the confidentiality of patients and their families as a sacred
trust and have therefore hidden names, genders, and settings,
combining stories and comments so that all identities have been
protected to the best of my ability. Should anyone identify with
any patient or family member it is most likely coincidence, and a
testament of the universality of these stories.

ISBN
978-1-03-911426-5 (Hardcover)
978-1-03-911425-8 (Paperback)
978-1-03-911427-2 (eBook)

1. PSYCHOLOGY, GRIEF & LOSS

Distributed to the trade by The Ingram Book Company

Table of Contents

About the cover photo: These images are taken from a sacred mandala I named "Dwelling in the Realm of Mortality." Painting a mandala is a complex, structured, mindfulness practice. For 14 months, I meditated on the Death Card from the tarot and painted daily as I wrote my dissertation while asking the question: What is the experience of counsellors who encounter mortality on a daily basis in the palliative care context?

This being human is a guest house.
Every morning a new arrival.

A joy, a depression, a meanness,
some momentary awareness comes
as an unexpected visitor.

Welcome and entertain them all!
Even if they are a crowd of sorrows
who violently sweep your house
empty of its furniture,
still, treat each guest honourably.
He may be clearing you out
for some new delight.

The dark thought, the shame, the malice,
meet them at the door laughing and invite them in.

Be grateful for whoever comes,
because each has been sent
as a guide from beyond.

Rumi

I am often asked what I will do when I retire. All I want, really, is to spend the rest of my life being kind.

This book is dedicated to Jane Johnston, who has inspired me by her way of being, to be a kinder more generous person.

BEGINNINGS:
What it means to work in palliative care

The Appointment

The disciple of a Sufi of Baghdad was sitting in the corner of an inn one day when he heard two figures talking. From what they said, he realized that one of them was the Angel of Death. The Angel was saying to his companion, "I have several calls to make during the next three weeks."

Terrified, the disciple concealed himself until the two had left. Then, applying his intelligence to the problem of how to cheat a possible call from Death, he decided that if he kept away from Baghdad, he should not be touched. From this reasoning, it was but a short step to hiring the fastest horse available and spurring it night and day towards the distant town of Samarkand. Meanwhile, Death met the Sufi teacher and they talked about various people. "And where is your disciple so-and-so?" asked Death. "He should be somewhere in this city, spending his time in contemplation, perhaps in a caravanserai," said the teacher. "Surprising," said the Angel, "because he is on my list. Yes, here it is: I have to collect him in four weeks' time at Samarkand, of all places." (Shah, 1993, p. 191)

You and I both know that we are going to die. Whether we embrace this knowledge, understand it, run from it, or pretend that it's not going to happen, we all have an appointment with death. After 20 years as a palliative care counsellor working at hospice, my appointment with death seems all too real.

What Shapes Us

When you are immersed in an occupation, it seems inevitable that you will develop heightened sensibilities associated with your work that will shape how you view the world, how you interact with your environment, and who you become as a person. For instance, if you are an architect, a photographer or an artist, when you walk down the street or are in a social situation, you will notice the lines of a building, the shapes of the landscape, or the play of light on people's faces. It's just natural that your attention will be drawn there. The time you have spent attuning yourself to light, shape and form has sharpened your awareness of a particular reality. In the case of a palliative care counsellor, what is the effect over time of being in the presence of death?

This question became the focus of my doctoral research. Through writing and reflecting, I came to appreciate the awe-inspiring, complex nature of my work and I realized that the anticipation of death has shaped everything about me—what I care about, what I fear, and my way of being in the world. But in conversation with others, it became apparent to me that, generally, even for people who work in the field, what counsellors do, why we do it, and the skill set that we use are either misunderstood or invisible.

Talking with a fellow education student about my work, she asked me, "Do you actually deal with death on a daily basis?" Perhaps the answer seems obvious to those of us who work in palliative care. Death permeates every aspect of our work. As professor at Athens University Danai Papadatou (2009) observed in her book, *In the Face of Death*, death is the unseen third party in every interaction. It is visibly, palpably present every day, and its effects spill over into time away from the work, because observing and interacting with those who are dying and bereaved automatically produces a questioning of life: How have we lived it? How are we living it? How will we live it?

Palliative Care

Encountering mortality in an environment where there is a network of people and systems to respond to the expectation that death is present, and where there is a set of values that connects these networks, is referred to as the "palliative care context." This context is different from encountering mortality in a hospital, on a battlefield, in someone's kitchen, or in a public place like a highway or a recreational area. It is different from experiencing death caused by a widespread disaster, such as a fire or an earthquake. Within a palliative care context, death is inevitable and will happen within a relatively short period of time. To address all of what this means, the treatment or care that we provide considers the needs of both the patient and his or her family.

Palliative care is a program of care that includes the physical space where all of the services are provided, supported by the philosophy of care. This care is based on a unique combination of values, attitudes and belief systems that are all reflected in how we connect and interact with patients and their families.

Papadatou (2009) identifies a number of beliefs that define palliative care. The first is an overarching acceptance that death is a natural part of life, and "that the focus of care for both patients and families is the experience of living with the awareness and reality of death" (p. 8). Caregivers demonstrate, through their way of being and relating, that encountering mortality is a profound experience that results in "networks of people who are changed forever as a result of loss" (p. 8).

A second belief is that holistic care must be provided by an interdisciplinary team. In palliative care, the interdisciplinary team works together to solve problems. The team must create synergy to be effective and sustainable: to provide holistic, individualistic, and seamless care to patients and families; and to recognize the contributions of each team member's knowledge and skill set. Though synergistic, each remains clearly identifiable as a doctor, nurse, counsellor or spiritual-care provider.

A third belief is that personal relationships with the dying and their families are both important and necessary. A powerful, authentic, human-to-human relationship is so essential to palliative care that it requires a system of support to be woven into the very fabric of an organization. Writing in the *American Journal of Hospice & Palliative Medicine* (1999), Maria DiTullio and Douglas McDonald noted that a reliance on relationships requires "a rare mixture of interpersonal skills, compassion, and professional acumen ... that constitutes the 'soul' of hospice" (p. 641). Of course, the values associated with how we connect with each other are supported differently in every context and organization, but it goes beyond that. DiTullio and MacDonald wrote that, in one study, for most of the palliative caregivers interviewed, "philosophical allegiance extends beyond a commitment to organizational mission and is wholly embraced as a personal philosophy of life" (p. 647).

Palliative Caregivers

Interestingly, a number of researchers have found that, for palliative caregivers, expectations commonly *match* the reality of hospice work, and when the caregivers find equilibrium between their internal and external resources and the demands of the job, those caregivers can experience a sense of wholeness (DiTullio & McDonald, 1999; Jones, 2005). So palliative care can become the stage on which personal values can be and often are enacted. I believe that this was true for me: personal values may be part of what accounts for how I related to my work as a counsellor.

When you are in this field, you can't help but think about every aspect of death, and as I neared retirement, I began to think about my legacy—what would be left after I was gone? I wanted to make a statement about my work. I wanted to leave an impression. And I also wanted to make the field more accessible to those who have not dwelt in the realm of death like I have.

There is another small but important detail: I have often been asked if I get paid to be a counsellor. I find this question a bit galling, after 23 years of formal education and 35 years of experience as a counsellor. For that reason, I feel a need to shed some light on the skill that it takes to do this work ... but it is so much more than that. I want to acknowledge the courage it takes, the willingness to walk into the unknown without a script, and the vulnerability we counsellors feel in allowing our own losses from the past and the possible losses in the future to appear in our imaginations over and over again, in order to understand what others are going through. It takes guts to face those we serve with all of our humanity—and not just as professionals with valuable information to offer. For counsellors in palliative care, there is no hiding behind a role. It's a profession that requires one to look long and deep into one's own soul. Through story, I hope to bring this quest to life.

As palliative care counsellors, we are called to enter into intensely emotional, often urgent situations, *every day*. We must immediately build some kind of rapport, and rather than give everything that we know—as in, a prescription for navigating death—we have to offer only the help that seems to be needed. So, we attempt to make an assessment, even though we may need to act or respond immediately. All this, while sorting through our own reactions, memories, fears and ambitions—which can be intrusive and distracting—in order to keep the focus on those who need our help. Self-reflection and self-knowledge are essential to the work of a counsellor, along with the constant practice of being present, which can be cultivated, but never fully attained.

Counsellors interact in a wholehearted, personal way in intimate moments with patients and their families, at a time of profound change. We can often positively affect a desperate situation, where vulnerable people feel completely overwhelmed on every level of their beings. Our ability to calm people, by listening and responding to what they have to say, and to convey deep compassion, may be why we are often described as "angels," or thought of as "special."

I think it is important to spend a moment exploring this concept, because it is such a common reaction when any palliative care staff member tells people for the first time that we work at hospice.

Being Special Versus Being of Service

For me, there is tension in accepting that I am special because I have done this work. The word actually makes me squirm. Why is that?

On reflection, I wonder if the discomfort has to do with my experience being considered weird when I was growing up, because I was interested in all that was hidden, protected and unspoken. Is this a question of identity, then? Perhaps I have an underlying fear that being drawn to the intensity and intimacy involved in caring for the dying and the bereaved reveals something "not quite right" about me, or, as a colleague put it, perhaps it means being special in a "creepy" way. Conversely, maybe the work reinforces and verifies that I am not weird, and that my way of being in the world is worthy of respect and honour, after all.

According to the *Oxford English Dictionary*, (2012) the word "special" derives from the Latin *specialis*, which means "specific, particular, individual or special" (np). Another meaning of the word "special" is related to palliative care work being specialized—that is, requiring knowledge and skill outside of what the ordinary person knows or does. We acquire those, as anyone does in whatever their field may be, through a combination of study and experience. There is no evaluative quality necessary here, simply the facts: we know more about this subject than most people do. On a practical level, having devoted ourselves to learning about palliative care because of a particular interest means that we are able to guide those who find themselves in the foreign territory of illness, death and bereavement.

Some counsellors feel grateful to have gained knowledge that has been useful in personal interactions with dying loved ones. Others appreciate that they have come to fear death less than they did before they were exposed to it so often. Our specialized knowledge provides an opportunity to know the secrets of the body, what can go wrong, how to be in the presence of suffering, and, at times, how to comfort those in pain.

In some ways, our specialness is ordinary, because everyone has something special to offer. One of my colleagues told me that she thinks that her accountant is a special kind of person. I had to laugh, when she went on to say,

> My God, if he didn't like his work, I might have to do my taxes!! And I think bus drivers are special people—that work looks to me to be so mind-numbingly boring, thank goodness they do it!! And what about the woman who sets rat traps in my house when I need them? She actually likes her work! She says she grew up on a farm and is drawn to her work. Wow, to me that is a special person. (Study Participant)

In my experience, palliative care counsellors do not generally think that they are better than others; we are just people who are happy, or perhaps just inclined, to do the work. We can appreciate that many people feel relief that we are willing to do it.

Another important reason that we may want to reject being deemed "special" is because it seems to imply that, because we have answered the call, there is something inherent in us that does not see or feel what other people experience. We know that that is not true, because if it were, it would negate our struggle to be present, and it would dismiss the discipline, the energy and the focus that we must find on a daily basis. It would deny our overriding desire to be of service for the good of humankind as a spiritual practice—and the way we value that service. I think where we differ from most people is that we have both the opportunity and the willingness to walk into this sacred, often frightening, fascinating, and enriching territory, while others are nudged by circumstance into the realm of death.

It often happens that, when we leave a family, we remark on what an "amazing job" they are doing, or we say to them, "I don't know how you do it." They often seem startled. One man I visited said, "I'm just doing what any loving person would do." Another family member said, "I can't imagine doing anything else." Family caregivers experience the same surprise and discomfort as we do when they are labelled "special." Although it can serve our ego, our goal is to be of service, not to be special.

Being of service, however, is not to be taken lightly. In this case, it required many years of formal education. But formal education was just the beginning. The focus of our work is really much more about the art rather than the science of navigating relations with the people we meet in a day; how we approach patients and their social networks, and how we interact with our colleagues who have different training, responsibilities and goals of care and, most importantly, different ways of being. We all have moments when we feel completely useless and have no idea how to connect in ways that are helpful, and other moments of pure brilliance when we make deep connections that obviously help tremendously, and of course, everything in between.

Being Present for My Own Story

Although it is clear from the literature that the key to providing good palliative care is the ability to be present, I've wondered what that really means. How do counsellors attempt to be present when, like everyone else, we have varying capacities to witness horrible sights and smells, to bear the most intense emotions, to struggle with ethical dilemmas, and to face spiritual and existential crises? Haunting images of tremendous suffering, memories of witnessing touching moments of profound love, and the joy of meeting the most interesting people have embedded themselves into our psyches. Some images can linger for decades.

Counsellors, like everyone else, have individual psychologies that make it difficult, if not impossible, to be present for some people, some situations and some emotions. What do we do when we don't want to be there, when what we want the most is to head for the hills?

The story that I am about to tell reveals some of the internal struggles that counsellors face, because it seems that we do not write much about our experiences in palliative care. I believe that knowing and understanding what we do, and how challenging it is, will be of interest to those who have wondered how or why anyone would do this work, or have themselves been drawn to the work. Along the way, I hope that readers will come to appreciate some of the nuances of counselling practice, as well as some possible responses to facing mortality.

Service Through Story

This book may be of interest to anyone who has ever wondered what it might be like to encounter death on a daily basis in a palliative care setting, or who has wondered what it would be like to encounter their own death, or the death of others. For some, the thought of interacting on an ongoing basis with the uncertainty and the emotional, physical and spiritual suffering associated with death seems frightening and overwhelming. Yet for others, or at other times of life, death can be welcomed and anticipated, almost a relief. Being present, not being present, living with the reality that we are all going to die, the visceral experience of coming face to face with death and grief—the desire to step closer and the equal desire to look away—can be confusing, creating waves of emotion that can be overwhelming to the psyche.

In my opinion, all in all, life as a palliative care counsellor is a wonderful, heart-warming, awesome job—despite many difficult, terrifying, gruesome times. In the telling of my story, I have attempted to communicate both the knowledge and the theory that underlie counsellors' formal training, while at the same time trying to demonstrate the creativity and skill with which we attend to our patients and their families. This requires us to pay attention to what is happening with others around us, and to attune our physical sensations and emotions, allowing for a sort of "third space" that observes both the internal and external happenings and makes comments or directs us, so that our hearts and our heads are aligned in harmony. The quality of our connection with others, and our work in general, depends on how well we are able to do this.

There is even some "third space" in this book: I have begun most of the chapters with a preface or lesson that can serve as a lens through which to view the story. These pieces reflect the academic training needed for the job. They may also provide contextual information that enriches the tale. As a whole, through weaving theory and practice, I hope that this book realistically reflects the job of a palliative care counsellor.

In all of it, it is important to me to be authentic, to portray the work and myself as accurately as possible, and to not romanticize or portray myself in any way other than how I really come across.

I begin by reflecting on the cultural directives of facing mortality which formed the basis for my own quest to wholeness—a quest that eventually led me to hospice. I then move into my personal story of my son Dante's death, in "Sacred Time." All of the names I used in this story are real, and the story itself is as it happened ... at least in my memory. This story will hopefully help the reader understand how my community inspired me to come forward to support those facing imminent death, either as patients or family members. Later, in "A Fate Worse Than Death," I tell the story of my mother's dementia and death as I remember them, although I have been purposefully vague when it comes to naming my sisters. Between and around those two chapters, I weave my personal story into the stories of the people whom I worked with and for, all within the palliative care context in my role as a counsellor, including one story in which my attendance at a conference as a professional overlapped with my personal losses.

In keeping with the genre of creative non-fiction, I have aimed in each story to come as close to the truth as is ethically possible, but, at least in some cases, I have significantly changed details to protect the identities of patients and their families. In other words, the stories are true, but not always factual. I have changed names and locations and created composites of stories and characters. Readers will find me working on the Palliative Care Crisis Team at what, for the purposes of this book, I have called "Meadowview Hospice." On that team, a nurse colleague and I responded to crisis calls from registered hospice patients and their families living in the community, or to follow-up calls on the in-patient unit.

It is my intention in this book to be scrupulous in attending to the sacred agreement of confidentiality, and my hope is that no trust has been broken in telling these stories. While it is possible—and even likely—that many readers will be able to imagine that the story being told is their own, each one is a combination of real events and is not about any specific person or people. Identification with the characters is simply a testimony to the universality of the themes.

CHAPTER ONE:
Hearing the call to hospice

How Culture Shapes Attitudes

Encountering mortality in the 1950s in Western Canada, where I grew up, was perhaps a different experience than it would have been in other parts of the country, other parts of the world, or today. Vestiges of dated social rules remain, and values of that time form the foundation of how we encounter mortality today. Attitudes that had perhaps served people through a challenging political era encouraged them to be "pleasant" and to maintain a "stiff upper lip" in the face of adversity. That "social directive" to not complain or speak about emotions at the risk of upsetting things also kept the realities of death and bereavement hidden from view, as unacceptable to "polite society."

For as long as I can remember, I have been fascinated by subjects that others do not want to talk about—religion, sexuality, underlying anxiety and tension, family secrets—as well as existential questions about life and death.

The first two encounters with mortality that I remember happened when I was about five years old. One involved my maternal grandfather, who lived with our family in a Vancouver suburb in Western Canada's version of 1950s Pleasantville. I was at a friend's house when her mother told me to go home immediately. Arriving at home on my bicycle moments later, I saw an ambulance parked in the driveway, lights flashing and doors open. My mother had covered her face, and her body was hunched over and heaving. My grandfather was lying on the stretcher, and I could see that his face was a strange grey colour. He was not moving. Was he dead? Standing alone on the lawn, I wondered, 'Did I just see a dead body?' No one told me directly that he had died. There was no mention of a funeral, although I know that one occurred.

Several years later, I asked my mother where my grandfather was buried. She told me that she didn't want to talk about it:it was too sad. When I said that I just wanted to take some daffodils to his grave, she gasped and began to cry, repeating more adamantly that it was too sad to talk about. Ten years later, sitting at the kitchen table with my parents and 21-year-old sister, I once again asked where my grandfather was buried. My sister burst into tears and ran out of the room in disgust, spitting at me,

"Why do you have to be so ... so morbid?" I still do not know where he is buried.

It seems as though my family culture—and perhaps the greater culture—was not prepared for a child's questions about death. As William Worden observed in his 1996 work, *Children and Grief: When a Parent Dies*: "Children repeatedly ask questions. When children are not given accurate information, they will create information to complete the story. Unfortunately, such information can be more frightening to children than what really happened" (p. 487). Lacking anyone to clarify my information, I believed that a box in a storage cupboard in the basement contained my grandfather's skull, stored there by my mother. It never occurred to me to ask my mother about it. Every time I had to walk past the cupboard to go to the piano, which had been moved into the place where my grandfather's bed used to be, the place where he had died, I ran past in fear. My parents could not understand why I suddenly did not want to practise the piano. It was only in passing conversation, many years later, that I realized that it could not have been my grandfather's skull in the box.

My second encounter with mortality involved a neighbour named Alice who took me to kindergarten. I heard that she had breast cancer, and I remember the whispers about her breast being removed. For some reason, I thought that it had been replaced with a wooden prosthesis.

I can still picture the imagined wooden carving: a perfect cone, banging against her scarred chest, filling the empty side of her bra. I speculated as to which one it was, looking for clues, rubbing up against her to see if I could feel the hard edge. Once again, it was only later that I realized that she had never had a wooden breast.

The secrecy created a sense of shame. I felt ashamed for wanting to know. This sense was reinforced a few years later, when I ran up the street to witness a child who had been hit by a car, being placed in an ambulance. I remember the rush of emotion—both fear and excitement—and the embarrassment of wanting to look. I was shooed away. I was beginning to understand that serious illness, injury and death were not talked about, and that people who wanted to talk about them were not okay. By the time some friends decided that it might be cool to dig up a pet turtle that we had buried, I was unable to look, afraid of what I might see, and I thought that they were being mean to even think of it.

And so, I arrived at estrangement from death, a stranger to death, or maybe just strange. It was clear that it was not socially acceptable to wonder about death or to ask questions, that my curiosity was painful to others, and that this and all other topics with an emotional charge were dangerous. It was easy as a child to then assume, from the responses up to that point, that people around me would crack if emotion was present. So, rather than be responsible for them coming undone, I cut off my own feelings and my sense of what it was to live life as a whole being.

My next encounter with death and serious illness was at age 14, when my paternal grandfather died. Shortly before he died, and after several years of awkward visits to a seniors' home that smelled strongly of urine and exposed me to an array of limp, white-haired people staring into space, I found out that my grandfather had contracted gangrene and had to have his leg amputated. I overheard conversations between my parents and refused to visit, fearing what a man without a leg might look like. By then I had developed a fear of sickness, hospitals, hospital equipment, doctors, and any disability, including—in fact, especially—anything associated with old age.

That left me particularly unequipped to deal with my own personal challenges when, at age 31, my father died within six months of receiving a terminal cancer diagnosis, my aunt died from a heart attack on a visit intended to console my grieving mother, and my brother died suddenly from a rare form of leukemia. All of this occurred within a five-month period, during which time my second child was born. Encountering mortality became unbearable, and I sank into despair. I was completely unable to process the overwhelming array of feelings, and there was no one to guide me through. I felt shame at being unable to "get over it," and I had a sense of stigma and self-consciousness, an irrational fear that maybe there was something inherently wrong with my family, as a group of people, for having so many awful things happen to us in such a short time.

With his article, "Living in the Liminal Spaces of Mortality," psychologist Martin Frommer (2005) helped me understand my fear of becoming known as a member of what I called the "bummer" family:

> Addressing one's relationship with death ... can feel fraught with uneasiness. People who dwell on their mortality are suspect. Culturally to do so is often experienced as crossing a boundary, breaking a taboo. And there are consequences: one runs the risk of being viewed as 'other,' labelled gloomy—a downer—or, in our own circles, imagined to be clinically depressed. The subject of mortality raises powerful anxiety, and our minds employ all manners of defence in an effort to shield us from a full awareness of our transience and its implications. pp. 479-498

Over the following 10 years, through the development of a supportive network of friends and improved relationships with my sisters, I was able to come to comprehend and assimilate the multiple deaths that I had experienced. Sensing what seemed like a lack of wholeness and having a desire to heal, I became a seeker by engaging in long-term, in-depth psychotherapy, meditation, prayer and reflection. Like Isis collecting the body of Osiris, I tried to gather and put back together my disjointed, disconnected pieces, in the hope that I would feel whole.

Nothing, however, prepared me for the death of my three-month-old son, Dante, from sudden infant death syndrome (SIDS) eight years later. It was by far the most difficult death that I have ever had to go through, and it was the event that had the most impact on my life. Surprisingly, and perhaps para-doxically, the time that I felt the most alone and vul-nerable was when I also felt the most connected and supported. The profound grief that I experienced was met by the equally profound loving presence of a wide network of friends, family, acquaintances and, in some cases, even strangers. Through their actions, they showed me that it is possible to make a space for and to be present for the intense, irre-versible, emotional, physical, intellectual, spiritual and social effects of encountering death.

Two aspects of this experience are particularly relevant to this book. The first was that the care offered by the people around me—the quality of their presence—afforded me a protected space in which to process the extreme, incapacitating grief that I felt. In her book, *The Four-Fold Way: Walking the*

Paths of the Warrior, Teacher, Healer, and Visionary, anthropologist Angeles Arrien (1993) teaches that "showing up" or "choosing to be present and visible" is recognized in many indigenous societies; it means to be able to bring our minds, emotions, spirits and physical beings to a situation: "When we choose to 'show up' energetically, with all four intelligences, we express the power of presence" (p. 23). I learned from my own experience when Dante died that when people "show up," it really does matter. Being on the receiving end of that presence clearly shaped me.

The second important aspect was an experience that I have rarely heard others talk about. In explaining that the "liminal recognition of mortality" can be met with ambivalence, Frommer (2005) described his clients' experiences as they remembered the events of September 2001: "It was a seemingly paradoxical experience that in the midst of intense anguish and grief, they felt an opening in themselves to an uncommon experience of connection with humanity. Some have since bemoaned the gradual fading of this capacity, coupled with a return to a more familiar self-state organized around denial of the human condition" (p. 487).

I can relate. Shortly after Dante's death, I had an extraordinary experience that words cannot adequately describe. What I can say is that, for a period of time, I became acutely aware of being alive. Every sensation was bright, clear—almost magnified.

Everything was peaceful and very beautiful. Being so close to death, so aware of the fragility of life, I saw how thin the veil is between life and death, and in the process, I experienced what can only be described as ecstasy. Looking back, I believe that I had this experience because I felt connected—to myself, to my own internal moment-to-moment experience, to my friends who offered a compassionate presence, and to the great cosmos that contains the mystery of life and death. Experiences such as this were often referred to by Carl Jung and identified by the writer Rudolph Otto in 1923 as "numinous." I saw clearly that life is intrinsically connected to death; they are inseparable. Most importantly, I realized that facing death can be an opportunity to open up to life.

Writing in 1957 about the therapeutic or healing experience in therapy, Carl Rogers, the founder of client-centred psychology, said that when a client has the direct experience of the therapist's acceptance, for whatever feeling is being expressed at the time, and, in whatever mode it is being expressed— through words, gestures or tears—the client will feel wholly accepted or "received." Having felt "received" by the people who surrounded me, I wanted to provide that same therapeutic experience to other bereaved people. Like an elder who has acquired wisdom and experience, I saw myself as having an important role in helping people find their own way through grief, by providing a safe space for them to express their powerful emotions and to explore what, for some, can seem like a dark and frightening place.

For many years, I opened my bereavement groups and my training workshops with a gender-neutral version of Judith Duerk's reflective question from her book, *Circle of Stones*:

> How might your life have been different if, as a young ... [person], there had been a place for you, a place where you could go to be among ... [elders] ... a place for you when you had feelings of darkness? And, if there had been an ... [elder], to be with you in your darkness, to be with you until you spoke ... spoke out your pain and anger and sorrow. ... So that, over the years, and companioned by the ... [elders] you learned to no longer fear your darkness, but to trust it ... to trust it as the place where you could meet your own deepest nature and give it voice. How might your life be different if you could trust your darkness ... could trust your own darkness? (p. 13)

Through my social network, with the help of those wise, kind, brave people who were able to show up, I found a home, a place where "I 'could trust my own darkness.'" By going into that darkness and reclaiming all of me, or my "whole" self, I wondered if wholeness, in the sense of being "restored or healed", needed to be expressed or manifested in order to be fully integrated into my being. Not only did I want to savour and repeat the sense of having gathered the parts, I wanted to understand how it had happened and to participate as a healing force in other people's lives in an ongoing way. I wondered if service might become both the path and the destination.

This quest, to find that which is whole/holy/sacred, led me to transpersonal psychology, and eventually to hospice. It was a search for an understanding of what it means to be wholly present in my own experience—not just for my own sense of being integrated, but to understand and connect with others and their experiences. It was also a quest to discover what it means to be human. Hospice held the promise that the profound effect of encountering mortality would be recognized, and my desire to be wholly present might be respected, valued and held sacred.

Hospice Is a Call to Wholeness

It is probably not surprising that my search for meaning and an authentic life would lead me to palliative care. But paradox abounds in encounters with mortality. Why would I think that I would find meaning in my life and live authentically by coming into contact with death?

According to the *Oxford English Dictionary*, (2012) the word "palliative" (palliate) comes from the Latin *palliatius* and means to "alleviate without curing," but it is also associated with the Latin *palliare*, "to cover with a cloak," or "to disguise," and *pallium*, "a cloak." In palliative medicine, this means that symptoms are masked by medication, but the cause of the disease is not significantly affected. Therefore, the expected course of the disease will continue, but the patient will not experience physical symptoms. The World Health Organization tells us that the term "palliative care" can be distinguished from "palliative medicine" by the values, attitudes and beliefs that allow for attending to emotional, spiritual and social needs.

Similarly, as a palliative care counsellor, I cannot and do not hope to cure a person of their suffering. Rather, I accept suffering by holding people with/in their suffering, by helping them to be able to better bear their pain through a compassionate presence, and by making space for emotions and spiritual experiences to be *un*covered, if that is what is required.

As a palliative care counsellor I anticipate many deaths—that is, anticipate in the sense of waiting for death. If I saw an average of 10 dying and/or bereaved people in a seven-hour workday, I have quite possibly interacted with more than 7,000

people. That's a lot of people—and a lot of death. Interactions with colleagues, and with patients and their social networks, occur as the patient lives through his or her last months, weeks, days and hours. There are various aspects to my role, including establishing relationships; helping clients explore, express or contain feelings; obtaining and processing information; and communicating. As a team member, I strive to find a balance between being a unique and freethinking individual, and a collaborative team member who is part of a cohesive team that patients and families can rely on and trust. It is important to me to cultivate a loving, calm and reassuring presence. My sincere desire is to connect—with my own experience, with others' experiences, and with the life force that is indescribable and unknowable.

In my role I am also called upon to witness death itself, which can occur peacefully, as expected, in a beautiful way that connects us to a force, nature, or spirit greater than ourselves—even if it is simply the realization that death is an inevitable part of life, something that people throughout history have been challenged to accept. At other times, death comes under extremely difficult, stressful, ugly circumstances that challenges every person present and causes me to wonder why life can be so painful, and why some people have to struggle so much. Writing in *Being and Time*, the philosopher Martin Heidegger (1953/1996) said that "we do not experience the dying of others in a genuine sense; we are at best always just 'there'" (p. 222).

In describing what it is like for nurses to witness their patients die, critical care nurse and scholar Pilar Camargo (2005) reflected upon her experience by saying:

> I can share my life, my dreams, my grief and all the things that join me with another person, but at the moment of death the word 'share' is left behind. We cannot delegate our death, for this moment just arrives. Where and when it arrives is impossible to know. Unable to share death, human beings share their lives. As a nurse, I just can be with Mr. Ricardo. I can share those last moments with him. I can rub his skin, control his vital signs, but I cannot die with him. I cannot feel what he is feeling now in those last moments. I am just a watcher. Although I am with him, at the same time, he is alone. As a nurse, I can cross death, but my experience is different from his experience. I could feel some kind of the same feeling when someday I die. None of us, however, can know what we will experience until we are actually dying ourselves. (pp. 8-9)

For counsellors, attending to the dying requires us to respond to what is asked of us in any given moment, and although there is much that we can anticipate, there are always aspects for which we cannot plan. Attending to the dying might involve holding a person's hand, speaking quietly, praying, meditating, or maintaining silence as a person takes his or her last breaths. It may mean a silent, solo vigil at the patient's side, or staying with a patient's family and friends, other hospice colleagues, or volunteers. It might mean standing, sitting, or kneeling at the bedside, in the corner of the room, at the foot of the bed, in the doorway, or it might involve comforting the dying person or his or her family. It might mean providing information or practical help. Sometimes it may mean simply being present. If I enter the space after the death had occurred, I may clean, straighten, wash or tidy the body and the surroundings, perhaps with family, but most often with a nurse. The work also extends into bereavement, creating a space for family and friends to continue to process the many losses triggered by the death.

At times, I meet death with compassion and a loving presence, and at other times, I feel fractured and disconnected—swinging between the extremes of this spectrum, moment to moment. Sometimes I am met in my attempt to connect, as others express a need or wish to connect with me, and other times, I do not. It is my desire to meet each circumstance with equal ease—both my own disconnection, and that of others.

Most people only deal with a few deaths during the course of their lives, so they can sometimes forget that we are all going to die. In palliative care, we can never forget: at work, encountering mortality happens continuously, over a long period of time. I can envision the process of connecting to and disconnecting from the reality of death as a spiral that takes me deeper and deeper into life, while at the same time moving me closer and closer to death. The spiral also moves through the paradoxes that are created as we approach and support death.

It is clear to me that my experiences in childhood, together with the deaths of a number of family members in rapid succession, followed by the death of my son Dante, created a profound sense of mission for me. My work as a hospice counsellor has been my world for the past 20 years.

CHAPTER TWO:
Sharing my own story

In his book *What Dying People Want*, (2002) palliative care physician Dr. David Kuhl writes that:

> Talking about dying is very difficult. We are afraid that talking about death beckons it. We all know death is inevitable; death fascinates and disturbs us; but we don't want it to happen. Maybe, we think, if we don't talk about death, death might not notice us. Maybe if we ignore death, we might delay or even elude it. (p.125)

Facing death prompts a spectrum of complicated responses that can range from relief and welcome, to fear and avoidance. It may be difficult to understand why people would choose to place themselves where death is inevitable and recurrent. When we were children and were asked what we wanted to be when we grew up, I'm fairly sure that none of us said, "I want to attend to the dying and bereaved." So how did we choose this occupation? Did life events play a part? Or is there something particular about our makeup? Did this occupation fill a need for employment, or does the work have a deeper meaning? What made us think that we could do this work, and why would we even want to?

When I polled my colleagues for my doctoral research, responses to these questions varied, but a common factor was the remembrance of a defining moment when each of us was called to palliative care. The call for me began after the death of my son, Dante, in 1992. This is how I remember it.

Sacred Time

It is Wednesday, a special day at school for my daughter Rosanna—a day when there is very little structure and the kids can bring things from home to share with the class. Rosanna has a new teacher named Alex. She wants to bring Dante to the class to show her teacher and friends her new baby brother. I nurse Dante at 7:30 that morning and tuck him back into bed so that I can get the other kids to school. I assure Rosanna that we will come as soon as Dante wakes up. Our plan is that Kim, our babysitter, will take Malcolm to his dental appointment so that I can go to the school with Dante.

When Dante doesn't wake, I decide that really, I should be the one to take Malcolm, as this is his first dental appointment. I leave Kim to pack up Dante and meet me at the school. After the appointment, I pull into the parking lot at the school and notice Rosanna sitting on the front steps. She runs up to the car and asks me what the emergency is. I look at her blankly. She has apparently phoned home to find out where we are, and Kim has told her that she can't talk because there is an emergency. I tell her that I will go home and get Dante and return shortly. Rosanna wants to come with me, but I say no, I'll check it out and return as soon as possible. I imagine that Kim has something cooking and is having a hard time managing both the baby and the boiling pots.

I calmly return to the car to drive the few short blocks to my house. When I turn the corner onto my street, I can see an ambulance parked outside of our house. The adrenaline begins to pump. I bolt into the driveway and see Kim on the front porch looking very worried. There are only two people home, and if it isn't Kim then it must be Dante. Oh my God. Dante. My whole body begins to numb. I'll never forget that feeling. I get out of the car and start shouting.

"What Kim, what is it?"

"It's Dante, they've taken him to the hospital."

An ambulance attendant comes over to me, puts her arm around my waist and moves me towards the ambulance as she speaks in soothing tones. Once I am in and we have pulled away, she says, "They've taken Dante to the hospital, and I'm going to take you there now."

It is like being in a movie, only played at slow speed. I say, "How is he?"

Then tentatively, "Is he dead?"

I'll never forget what she says next.

"I'll be honest with you. It doesn't look good."

It all seems so unreal.

It takes forever to travel the few blocks to Emergency. I run through the sliding double doors and see Bruce. We are led into a tiny room. He tells me that the Emergency crew is trying to revive Dante, but that he has seen him and he is definitely dead. Shaking his head, he says, "We don't want them to revive him, he'd be too brain damaged."

I pick up the phone and call my dear friend and midwife, Luba. Miraculously, she answers. I say, "Luba we're at the hospital. We think Dante is dead."

She says she'll be right over.

We sit in silence, waiting for we don't know what. The doctor comes in after what seems like a really long time and tells us that there was nothing they could do; our son is dead. Bruce and I cry together through a curtain of unreality.

I phone my sister Karen, in Vancouver. She is leaving on a cruise in two hours. I leave a message.

"Karen don't go. Dante has died and I need you. I know this is hard for you, but I really need you. Don't disappear on me."

Then I phone Elayne and Marion. We have been meeting once a week for dinner at Marion's restaurant, sharing intimacies. Each of us having four children is one of the bonds that connects us. I tell them that I am at the hospital and that Dante has died. Then I phone home, because Kim has been left there with Malcolm, not knowing what is going on. I tell her that Dante has been pronounced dead. She will bring Malcolm over right away.

I turn to Bruce and say, "I know people split up when something like this happens. I don't want that to happen to us."

He doesn't think that will happen to us. His worry is that he will be expected to be strong. I assure him that that is not what I want.

Luba arrives. I want to be with Dante, but I'm afraid to see him, I don't know what to expect. She goes and looks at him for me and tells me that he looks lovely, just very pale. She warns me that he has tubes up his nose. We are taken to an Emergency treatment room. Dante is wrapped in a big hospital blanket, so tiny on a huge steel table. I begin to scream, stamping my feet in anger. This I alternate with putting my arms around him, kissing him and wailing,

"Don't go, I love you, you are so beautiful."

I know that he's gone, and there's nothing that I can do about it.

Luba asks me if I want her to go and get the kids before school is out for the day. We don't want Kim to be left with telling them the news. She leaves in a taxi. Oh, my poor babies. A nurse comes and tells us that we can't stay. I am definitely not going anywhere without Dante. She leaves, and I take off Dante's little pink sleeper. I want to see his beautiful body. He is still warm, but he is losing colour quickly. I hold his toes, as I have always done with my children, trying to keep them warm. This time, his little toes are not going to warm up. His fingertips are blue where his blood has pooled. I can't believe this is happening.

Meanwhile, Luba has called a cab, not realizing that she has no money with her. She tells the driver that she is on her way to do the most difficult thing she has ever had to do. She explains that she will have to tell two children that their baby brother has died. The driver refuses payment and waits outside while she goes in, so he can bring them all back to the hospital. Luba explains to the principal what has happened, and the principal goes to get the children. Ryley must have intuited something, because when he leaves the classroom, he asks the principal if he should get some tissues.

Luba comes back with Ryley and Rosanna, who are crying. Kim arrives with Malcolm. Now we are back in the teeny room off Emergency. While we talk, Luba arranges for Dante to be taken to a larger room, where the kids can be with him and we won't be hurried along. We ask the kids if they are ready to see him. Ryley is sure that he isn't. Rosanna says maybe, and Malcolm wants to. Kim and I take Malcolm in. He touches him and we all cry. I can only imagine what Kim has been through and what this is like for her. Soon Rosanna joins us. She keeps her distance.

I am sitting on a table holding Dante's little body. I am fairly calm at this point, and I motion for her to come closer. I tell her that he looks beautiful. She takes him from me and holds him closely to her. She is crying softly, privately, the way Rosanna does things. She kisses him, hands him back to me and goes out with Luba. I hand Dante to Bruce and go back to speak with Ryley, who doesn't want to come in. I encourage him and he agrees, tentatively approaching the small bundle. He lifts Dante's fingers and lightly touches his skin. He doesn't want to stay.

When Bruce and I return to the small family room, Ryley and Rosanna are huddled together on the couch with Luba's arm around them. Malcolm is curled in Kim's lap, head nuzzled under her chin. We tell them that this is going to be a really hard time. We explain that we are all going to experience a lot of emotions, and that it is important that we are each allowed to handle the situation in our own way. We need to be really respectful of each other.

We tell them that they may feel like crying, but they also may not. We assure them that whatever they feel is just fine. Ryley says that it is really hard for Rosanna and him because they are not used to seeing us cry so much, and they don't like it. We say that we can understand that.

Then Ryley says, "I don't know about you, but I'm going to go home and escape into fantasy," meaning his science fiction novels. We say that is fine, if that is what you need to do, go for it. Kim leaves with all three of them.

I turn to Bruce when they leave and say, "I sure hope that I can make some meaning out of this, because right now it sure doesn't make any sense."

At some point, my friends Elayne, Marion and Eileen have arrived. We gather around the table where Dante is, stroking him and crying. I keep saying, "Look at him, he's so beautiful, he's so perfect, I don't want him to go, I love him, look how beautiful my baby is."

Michael, the doctor who delivered Dante, arrives at about the same time as the coroner. They say that they have to do an autopsy.

"No way," I say. "He's my baby, and you can't cut into him."

I know that I sound hysterical, and that is exactly how I feel. Luba says that although it seems awful and not very relevant right now, it might be important later to know exactly what he died of, just so we won't be left wondering.

I want to take him home, but they say I can't until the coroner is through. I didn't know that his body didn't belong to me. I am feeling that control is slipping away. There is also a detective there, asking us questions about the circumstances surrounding his death. I've worked as a child protection social worker, and although rationally I understand why he is there, it feels like they are bordering on being really offensive. I take deep breaths and I tell myself, 'He's just doing his job, try to be rational'.

There are subtle messages coming from the staff, urging us to leave. Luba keeps putting them off. Seven hours have passed. The coroner's office is going to take Dante's body to another hospital, and we are just waiting for them to come and get him. There is nothing more that I can do. There just isn't any point staying with him, and yet it seems so wrong to leave him. Elayne, Marion and Luba are Jewish, so they start to sing the songs for the dead, promising me that they will stay with him until the attendants take him away. Eileen comes with me.

I have never done anything as difficult in my life, as walking away from that hospital. Every bone in my body wants to stay. I know that they are going to put my precious son in a drawer. How could it be that just hours before, I had attended every need of his little body, wiping his little bottom, feeding him, laughing with him, taking such good care of him ... and now they are going to put him in a cold drawer. Eileen half walks, half carries me out. I ask her several times, "Eileen, would you leave him if it was your baby? Would you leave him all by himself?"

I feel torn apart, ravaged, the Scarecrow in *The Wizard of Oz*, ripped in little pieces by the flying monkeys.

When we get home, there are several casseroles and some muffins, and a note from David and Vicki that says, "This is so unfair. There can't be a God."

I don't really remember what happens in the next few hours, except that I feel sick to my stomach and I cry a lot. My sister Karen calls and says that she will be right over. She does come later that night, and so does my sister Lynda. My youngest sister Diane calls, and we cry and cry together. Diane has just left that morning with her first child, who is Dante's age. We were going to grow our babies together. I tell her not to come yet, and to make sure that mom doesn't come either.

My mom phones. I have been fighting with my mother for the last year. We have been trying to resolve it through letter writing, but it is far from finished. I come to the phone and she bursts into tears, saying, "I can't believe this is happening to me."

'No mom', I'm thinking, 'this is happening to me. It's my baby who died'.

"What have I done to deserve this," she went on. "First my husband, then my son, and now Dante. Am I cursed?"

I know that I'm being selfish and stubborn, but there is so much history that has to do with my perception that mom sees no one but herself. I have been there for her and taken care of her emotional needs for far too long, that this just seems too typical. I can see where the conversation is going to go, so I say, "Mom, I'm feeling a little overwhelmed right now. Do you think I could talk to you a little bit later? Don't come yet. I need some time."

"Of course," she says, "anything that I can do for you. I wish I could give my life so Dante could live."

I say good-bye. My friend Vicki must have been there, because I'm sure that I remember her giving me strokes for setting limits with my mother.

I don't know where Kim is. Kim is our beloved friend. She lives in a suite downstairs. She is a remarkable young woman of 23, more than a friend. She is more like a daughter, but also like a caring mother, and she loves my children as much as I do. We all adore her. She and her boyfriend Josh attended Dante's birth, and we asked them to be his godparents.

At some point, Kim comes upstairs and tells me what happened that morning. After I left, she suddenly had a feeling that she should check on Dante. She went upstairs and found him still and pale. When she realized that he wasn't breathing, she panicked, lifted him up immediately and started CPR. At the same time, she ran to our bedroom and, with one movement, wiped her arm across the bedside table, clearing it of everything. She laid Dante on the table, screaming in frustration at her hair falling in her face. Keeping her lips over his, breathing air into his still lungs, she managed to dial 911. They instructed her to keep up her efforts until the ambulance could get here. Time slowed, and she tells me that it was absolutely horrendous waiting for them to arrive.

When they finally did come, they pushed her out of the way and took over. She was left to stand helplessly watching. The only thing she could think to do was to phone Bruce at work and hysterically tell him to come home. He arrived home and left with the first ambulance, leaving Kim with nothing to do but wait for me to come home. When I finally arrived and then left for the hospital, she and Malcolm curled up on the couch in tears until the police arrived to ask her questions. I feel so sorry that she has had to go through this—she seems so young. I reassure her that she is not to blame in any way. Then she says that she is only glad that she could save me some small measure of pain by finding him, and that she is happy that she could do that for me. I love her so much.

We sit around late into the night. There is a lot of crying. Eventually it is time for bed, but I don't want to face the night, because I haven't forgotten that terrible feeling I had when my dad died, the one when you wake up and remember. I lie on the couch and listen to Bach's *Requiem Mass*. As the new day dawns, I go down to Kim's apartment and ask if I can sleep with her. Josh is there, so they both move over and I crawl in. Kim holds me while I cry myself to sleep. Unfortunately, I just can't rest for very long.

By the next day, my breasts have filled with milk and have really begun to hurt. My friends go to the Chinese herbalist and get me herbs and other disgusting things like dried locusts and buggy-looking objects to use as teas and poultices to dry up my breast milk. There I am, always struggling to establish my milk supply so that I have enough for my babies, and now I'm trying to get it to go away. My breasts are bursting, crying milk tears. There is something pathetic about squeezing milk down the drain.

My neighbour Melanie comes over to see if Emma and Charlotte, known collectively as "the girls," can come over to play with Malcolm. Standing at the front door, I cannot take in her words. "What's the matter?" she asks in alarm.

"Didn't you hear what happened?"

She looks surprised. We are frozen in time together for a few seconds, as I try to find the words. "Dante died yesterday morning."

She flings her arms around me and cries, one mother to another.

There are a lot of phone calls that day. Elayne and Marion sort of move in. Even though they each have four children of their own, as does my other friend Eileen, who is also there, they somehow manage to keep my house spotless and make warm, nourishing meals, beautiful sit-down meals for everyone who has gathered.

Vicki and David, fellow therapists, take lists of clients and cancel appointments until further notice. I don't want to burden my clients with this information, and I don't want them to feel that they have to take care of me. Vicki will assure them that I am in good hands and doing well.

Hours pass. We talk to Nick and Cynthia in Seattle. Cynthia is a Unitarian minister and agrees to be the celebrant for Dante's funeral. I cling to Dante's special teddy bear that my sister Karen gave him. Our friends do not leave our side. Elayne and Marion have established a routine of hot and cold compresses on my breasts, while urging me to drink the foul teas. They lead me to the tub, dress me, get me tissues, feed me, comfort me, and talk with me. It is like being a little baby and having every need anticipated. On some very deep level, I feel like I am being cared for in a way that I have never experienced before. Bruce experiences their care in the same way, like we are being healed deep inside of ourselves.

Malcolm wants me, and no one else, to pick him up from preschool, so Karen drives me. I'm standing on the steps of this yuppy preschool when I notice that I have on Kim's long underwear that has been dyed blue and has no elastic at the waist, with Bruce's neon orange and black T-shirt, clutching

Dante's teddy bear. I say to myself, 'Looking back on this. I'm probably going to feel really embarrassed'. But at this particular moment, I just don't care.

Rosanna and Ryley go to friends' houses. They don't like to hear us cry. Later, Rosanna tells me that she doesn't understand why people came and didn't try to cheer us up. It doesn't make sense to her that they would just let us cry. Malcolm pretty much moves in with his friends across the street.

One night, Bruce's men's group comes over to the house. These men have been meeting weekly for 20 years. Together they have supported each other through marriages, first houses, first children, teenage traumas, the death of parents—all kinds of life passages. Bruce sits on the couch, the men on either side of him, each touching some part of his body, stroking him. He begins to cry. He sits for the next two hours, crying and crying, nobody saying anything. For some reason it reminds me of Michelangelo's *Pietà*. The rest of us sit in the kitchen or go for walks.

We drink a lot of brandy. Someone from the men's group is at our house all day, from first thing in the morning until we go to bed at night. Neighbours and friends send a lot of food. My friends and sisters take care of everything.

Bruce and I decide to have a wake on Friday night. We make a list of people we want to be with, and Kim phones and invites them. I insist that Dante's body be brought home. Bruce says he's sure that they won't let us. There is subtle pressure not to do it. I get angry and say that I have three very assertive friends, Luba being one of them, and if they can't make the hospital release his body, no one can. They all exchange glances. They say that they can try. I get the distinct feeling that they are humouring me.

I'm in my bedroom with my friends, who seem concerned about the children seeing Dante's dead body. It is suggested that there is symbolism in simply having his empty bed. For me, it is important that things be kept real. I talk with Cynthia, our minister friend in Seattle. I tell her that people seem to have a problem with me bringing Dante home. She is really supportive and encourages me to do what is right for me. She reassures me that I am not being weird.

Later, I talk to Bruce. He seems angry with me. "This is going to be heavy—do you really think that you can handle it?"

"Yes," I say, looking him straight in the eye. "I want to have Dante with me."

He pauses.

"Maybe it's me that can't handle it. It scares me, it's too much feeling."

"I know," I say, my voice softening. I really love him in this moment.

I can't sleep. I stay up all night on the couch listening to music. We have set up a little table in the study with pictures of Dante's birth, of the kids walking with Dante, Dante in his little chair. We don't have nearly enough pictures. Of course, we had thought that there was all the time in the world to take more. We have lit the angel candles, and there are lots of flowers. There is a feeling of sacred space.

At about five o'clock in the morning, I go down to Kim's apartment and knock. She comes to the door naked, eyes only half opened. I say, "Kim I can't sleep. Do you want to go for a walk?"

She says, "Sure," with the enthusiasm only Kim can show after being woken out of a deep sleep. We head down to the beach. The sun is up and there is a huge rainbow that touches both horizons. We wonder if it is a sign from Dante, telling us that he is okay.

We talk about what happened. Poor Kim, she will live with this memory for a long time—trying to resuscitate a dead baby. To me, the image is horrible. Then having to deal with the police all by herself. It's a lot for a young woman.

I go home and find that there is no coffee. It's only seven o'clock, but I figure that our neighbours Melanie and Gordon will be up, so I go across the street. They are up, and they pour coffee into me, glad to be of help. We talk about how Malcolm is doing, and how the girls are taking it. Melanie has told them that Dante is with Jesus, in the sky. Somehow, Malcolm thinks that she has said "Mr. Jesus," so from then on, he tells people that his brother lives with Mr. Jesus in the sky. One time, about a month later, while having a bath, he wrinkles his brow and says "Is Dante really with Mr. Jesus?"

"Well some people think that."

"Do you?"

"No Malcolm, I don't, but it's still a nice thought. I would rather think of him flying free, past the sun, and all around the moon and stars."

He doesn't mention Mr. Jesus again.

On Friday, the kids come home from school while I am lying down. My mother is coming. Diane has arrived with her baby, Laiya. I cry. I hold her, but it's too painful. I feel jealous. I don't want to, but I just do. Diane understands.

My friends come over and lie down with me. I am dreading my mother coming. I can't take care of her. Vicki assures me that my friends will talk to her. Vicki holds me, and I feel safe. When my mom comes, it isn't as bad as I had imagined it might be. She keeps her distance.

Ryley comes into my room. I ask, "Ryley, how are you doing?"

"Okay," he says. "I don't feel like crying, though."

I reassure him that that is normal. I ask him how he's feeling about Dante being brought home for the wake. He says that he doesn't want to hurt my feelings, so he's not going to tell me. I say that it's okay, he doesn't have to protect me—I can take it. He takes a deep breath and says, "I understand that you have a need to be with Dante—I really understand that—but frankly, it disgusts me to see you holding a dead baby. I find it gross. My friend Quinn understands. I've talked to him about it and he agrees."

I tell him I'm really glad that he has told me this, and that I do understand how he could feel that way. He then goes on to say that, while he knows that you can't put grief on a scale, if you could, I would be way at the top, and then dad, and then maybe Rosanna. He would put himself far down the list; he just isn't feeling much. I tell him again how much I appreciate his honesty, and that I don't expect him to feel what I am feeling. I know that it is different to be a mother than a brother, and that he has had his own relationship with Dante, so of course he will feel differently. He reiterates how hard it is for him and Rosanna to see us crying, because he is used to us being the perfect parents ... not that crying makes you imperfect, it is just that usually we handle things pretty well. He says that he isn't looking forward to the wake and he probably won't stay. I say that is fine with me.

Rosanna, who is eight years old, and her nine-year-old cousin Jeff take all of their money and go shopping. They bring Bruce and I presents from the store, so that we won't be sad. They give us cards that they have made for us with mountains, rainbows and suns that say, "Be Happy." Such sweetness!

Later that night is pretty hard to describe. It is magical, it is profound, it changes everybody who is there. We have prepared the study, putting a pink tablecloth on the desk, tons of flowers and candles, and Dante's little basket with the velour quilt I had made for him. The men from the funeral home bring his body, and we lay it in his basket, all wrapped up. He has a bonnet on to cover the traces of the autopsy. Luba checks for me before I see him, to make sure that we are not going to see anything ugly, since I can be very squeamish about these sorts of things.

When I walk in and see him, I feel strangely exhilarated. Bruce feels it too. Dante is so beautiful, and it feels so right to have him home with us, one last time. We stay with him for what must be a long time, because when we come out, all of our friends are there—family and close friends, maybe 30 people altogether. We have asked that people bring something to share. I am holding Dante, seated on the floor.

The first person to share is a friend of Bruce's, Doug. I don't know him that well. He had gone for a walk that day and been thinking about all the wonderful things that Dante is going to miss. He is never going to run on the sand, so Doug brought him a box of sand. He is never going to chase falling leaves or skip rocks or enjoy all the pleasures of nature. Doug brought them to him, all wrapped up in little boxes. I am so deeply touched by what this man says. I cry and cry, rocking Dante's body.

On either side of me sit Casey and Lenni, two nine-year-old friends of Rosanna's, who have been around Dante a lot. They each hold one of his hands and croon to him. They lean on me, crying. It is good to have them there, so full of life. I notice Ryley there for a while, leaning against his friend Quinn. I haven't seen Rosanna since we started. I had noticed her earlier, dressed up in a formal dress of mine, then covered with a raincoat, holding an umbrella. She looked like the clothes were there to protect her. It was all too much for her, so she apparently sat out on the lawn by herself.

Everybody says something. Kulli, brings a baby hockey stick. Her son Eric had been going to teach Dante how to play hockey. It touches me to see how open she is. My Jewish friends sing "Kaddish," a hymn of praise, and Eileen sings a song in Latin, reflecting her Catholicism. My brother-in-law has written a poem. Kim talks about Dante's birth, and how our family had so much to offer him, how loved he had been. Everyone participates in one way or another.

Bruce takes Dante in his arms, and the men's group gathers around him and talks about what a wonderful father he is. John tells us about going to his mother's garden and picking a dead rose for Dante, despite his mother's protests. He goes on about getting in touch with a little part of him that has been dead for a long time, and how he wants to reclaim that part of himself.

An old friend, who has travelled to be here with me, tells us that she had been talking about Dante's death with her mother. Her mother then began to tell her, for the first time, about the two babies she had had, who had died. They had been able to cry about those babies together. Vicki brings a book by Robert Munsch, *Love You Forever*, the same book we had brought to her when she had Noah. My brother-in-law Danny talks about looking after Dante for an afternoon while I took the other kids to *Les Misérables*. He talks about Dante's fuzzy head, and the way he had smelled. We sing songs and cry and stroke Dante. We all vow to cherish the people we love while they are here, especially our children. We are all wide open. Finally, when everyone has spoken, we sing," Go Now in Peace," the song we sing in church when the children leave.

What means the most to me is that the people who I truly love are not afraid to deal with the intensity, with the depth of the feelings that the occasion evokes. I feel that my friends have met my pain. They have stretched themselves because they care about Bruce and me. I am so grateful for the love that surrounds me. I realize that it really is my own ability to face the truth that has guided the way. Dante is a divine presence in my life. His life has been a precious, beautiful gift. A gift that I had only begun to unwrap. I don't really know what is in store for me now. What I do know is that I have been profoundly touched by divine love. My love for Dante made this possible. I also know that I want to spend my time wisely. I want to reach out and be with other people in a new way—a way that allows my creative spirit to shine and allows other people to be touched by the light.

CHAPTER THREE:
Counsellors find being present challenging

The Physicality of Death

Although by the World Health Organization's definition, palliative care addresses psychosocial issues, not every palliative care organization employs a psychosocial specialist, such as a counsellor, psychologist, or social worker. The hospice at which I work—which I have given the pseudonym "Meadowview"—has a psychosocial team of about 20 members. Our numbers alone create a constant reminder of the psychosocial aspects of palliative care, and the fact that our leader sits at the management table, providing a strong voice for psychosocial interests, reflects the importance of our role.

There are a number of different areas of work for counsellors at Meadowview. Among them is the Palliative Care Crisis Team, or PCCT, which operates seven days a week, 24 hours a day. I worked on this team. The PCCT is made up of a counsellor-nurse team and is supported by a physician who is available to us 24 hours a day by phone and, if necessary, in person. I interpret this configuration as a statement and acknowledgment by the organization that psychosocial care is inextricable from physical care, and is therefore best provided by an interdisciplinary team.

In the following story, I introduce the counsellor and nurse who make up the PCCT team, and our community partner, the home care nurse. I also highlight an issue with which many counsellors struggle when they first arrive at hospice.

I should say that my previous training was in social work. There were no courses in hospital work or palliative care. Instead, I learned about the child welfare system, parole, sexual abuse, and family counselling. At the Master's level, I focused on transpersonal care, which is where spirituality and psychology meet. Although these areas are full of grief and loss, none dealt with the physicality of death.

A Home Visit

My nurse colleague receives a call from the home care nurse that Mrs. White's condition is changing and a route change is required, as she is now too weak to swallow pills. She needs her medicine delivered in liquid form under her tongue, or by a small needle under her skin. We arrive at the house and go into Mrs. White's bedroom where she is neatly tucked into bed. Cathy, the home care nurse, is seated at the bedside, holding Mrs. White's hand and leaning into the bed towards her. Cathy asks me if I will take over for her, gesturing with a shrug towards Mrs. White. I notice the hearing aids resting on the bedside table at the same time Cathy says to Mrs. White in a tender voice, "Mrs. White, I'm going to take my hand away, but someone else is here."

I say to Cathy, "Is she holding your hand?"

"Oh yes, she's holding it."

I am wondering if Mrs. White will welcome my touch. I feel warmth for Cathy because she appears to feel comfortable and so caring towards Mrs. White. She wants to hold Mrs. White's hand—she wants Mrs. White to know that someone is here caring for her. Cathy has her hand placed under Mrs. White's hand, so that Mrs. White can be in control; she can move her hand away if she wants to. This is what we have been taught to do. I want Cathy to stay, so that I can talk to the caregiver. I feel better able to talk or listen than to just "be." I feel no connection to Mrs. White, and I don't want to touch her dry and papery hand, but I don't want Cathy to think badly of me, to think that I am uncaring. Am

I uncaring? Cathy has shown me that Mrs. White is worthy of attention, of tenderness, of the intimacy of touch. Her gaze creates a bridge that takes me from the edges of the room, where I want to be, to taking a seat beside Mrs. White. I place my hand under hers. It is soft, dry and unmoving. Because I don't want to hold her hand, my hand is not savouring her touch. I don't lean my skin into hers, but rather hold it stiffly, making as little contact as I can manage. My imagination wanders as I dissociate from what is happening.

I wonder what it must be like to lie there, unable to hear, and too weak to open my eyes. I visualize myself in a small, light body. Immediately I feel vulnerable ... I wonder if she is in a state of trust, just lying there. She certainly is in a position to need to trust, but to trust, she would need to surrender. Maybe she had no choice but to surrender. I don't really know what is happening inside of her. I can only imagine what it might be like for me, with the experience that I have now. What would it be like to outlive a lifetime partner by 20 years? I see my husband in a coffin, me crying at his side. I see myself bravely going on to try to create a life by myself. And then I see myself getting some diagnosis, having to rely solely on my family and professionals to care for me.

A change in Mrs. White's breathing brings me back to her side. She has my attention. I lean towards her and make a slight adjustment, so that the palm of my hand touches the palm of her hand.

CHAPTER FOUR:
Being a counsellor requires empathy

A Call to An Alternate World

Why are people called to become palliative caregivers? According to psychologist and York University professor Ami Rokach (2005), "Many of those who help others do so because they genuinely care. They have deep compassion for the suffering of the dying and want to contribute in easing their pain" (p. 325-332). Many look upon this work as a genuine calling. Eve Joseph (2010) a Victoria, B.C. hospice counsellor for 20 years, ends a touching exploration of her experience in palliative care with words that speak of that same sense:

> For a long time, it was not just work; it was a calling. Not a religious call, although one can't do the work without

a deep sense of the mystery that surrounds the dying; rather, it was the thing
I did that made me feel most alive. Like
writing poetry. Hopkins referred to the
state of being aware, responsive, and
open as the taste of the self. A state, paradoxically, in which we are fully present
at the same time we disappear. To work
with the dying was to enter the darkness
without a map of the way home. It was
to merge, briefly, with something greater
than ourselves; to accompany them as
far as possible and to stand alone under
the stars they disappeared into. (p. 5-12)

Joseph observes a remarkable paradox: that a
palliative care counsellor experiences working with
the dying as "the thing that I did that made me feel
most alive." Hers was not an experience of standing
on the edge looking in, but rather her own powerful experience of wonder at what it means to live
and die.

In my doctoral research, I asked my colleagues
how they came to work at hospice. For one, it
began as a simple need to get a job, but it quickly
became an appreciation of the need to interact
authentically and intimately. The initial glimpse of
a different reality—one in which interactions with
others are loving, extending beyond the personal to
a visceral sense of unity—provided a sense of being

deeply connected to all of life. The regular masks and personas that people so often don in social situations fall away in the face of death. It seems natural then, in this setting, to arrive as ourselves, which naturally, effortlessly brings about a delightful, surprising ability; a willingness to welcome the other, in whatever form it comes.

Another colleague described a sense of "being love" rather than "being loving"; a sense of uncovering, a way of remembering what was always right there in her very nature:

> I feel intensely present in the unfolding of the moment—all senses wide open; deeply engaged, attentive and curious; non-attached—to outcome, people's decisions, what will happen ... —but not detached; willingness—to feel and be moved by life; grounded; compassionate; open-hearted—literally open/ spacious in the centre chest; empty/spacious/still—like an enormous container in which the experience of connecting is unfolding; and yet full—vibrant/ humming. There is a timelessness. In these "experiences" there is the sense of the particular beingness of the one meeting the particular beingness of the other "underneath" social construction—roles, status, gender, race,

etc.—and recognizing/knowing itself as beingness. For me, there is a sense of sacredness and deep respect here—a meditative, devotional stance in the world within which my training and skills are employed.

The call to the realm of the dying is a dawning awareness that there might be a different way to encounter mortality. Service calls to us by offering a hope that caring for the dying and bereaved will teach us something about how to live.

Being called to the realm of death is to be pulled out of the everydayness of life, a willingness to be off-balance, to have our sense of safety and famil-iarity challenged, to have the comfort of thinking that we know how it is, constantly disrupted. The call is to surrender to uncertainty, change and dis-comfort. This was the draw for another counsellor, who said that she had always been attracted to that which is outside normal experience. She said that she wanted to be awake, alert. She liked to be the "stranger living on the edge." She was not interested in "the realm of normal." She said that the sick are isolated in leper colonies, isolation wards, support groups, palliative care units, away from "domestic reality," and to heed the call of service was to follow the dying to "the outskirts of society."

On those outskirts, in one particular week, for instance, there were 15 deaths ... too many too fast to really know anyone or even remember their names. Continuing, the counsellor said, "[A]ll that remains are impressions: flickers of conversations, the colour of one daughter's hair, a tea cup held like an urgent promise, a photo of youth propped next to the bed. In the moment of being with that dying person and his or her family and friends, there can be a shock of intimacy, a connection that is real and mysterious. That, in itself, feels like something that happens outside of the centre. I am not seeking anything—I am not looking for a date or a job—I am only there to be present and, hopefully, useful. I have no expectation of a future with any of these people—everything is focused on this moment. This is not an exchange—I am not a neighbour who is offering a casserole to a widow knowing that someone else might do this for my husband when I die. This is a blessing pulled out of us." The call to the realm of death is a call to an alternate world, a world outside day-to-day routines, a world where the shock of death brought her into the moment— no plan, no agenda, no control. For this particular counsellor, when she is at her best, she says her "work is a prayer."

How do we live out the promise of a different way of being? Is it possible to maintain that desire, that commitment? In coming to hospice, there is a feeling of uneasiness, uncertainty, self-doubt about whether we can provide all of what caring for the dying and bereaved asks of us. We ask ourselves:

will we be able to sustain caring through what my colleague describes as the "depth, heaviness, and messiness of people's sorrow and despair"? There are challenges in turning towards death, even when we have the desire and the willingness to do so. What is it like to have D/death arrive at our doorstep every day?

For many of us, connecting deeply with those we serve can be a double-edged sword. Strongly identifying with the patient through our imaginations, for instance, helps us understand another's experience. But it can also create anxiety and stress to constantly envision ourselves as a patient, fading away, suffering physically, mentally and spiritually, or as a family member witnessing someone we love declining into oblivion. However, this identification also allows us to empathize. This, in turn, makes us appreciate our own health and leads to a sense of urgency to acknowledge and appreciate our own good fortune, as in the following story about Christine.

Sunday Dinner

The nurse, Kelly, and I arrive at the home of Christine. She has been admitted and discharged from our team a number of times, so I have seen her before, usually when she has been in an extreme pain crisis. We did an extensive evaluation on a previous visit, and today we are checking to see how she is doing, mentally, physically, socially, emotionally and spiritually since our team saw her yesterday. It often takes about five days to settle a person's physical symptoms—usually pain, nausea, and/or shortness of breath—to an acceptable level. Our team will stay involved until the symptoms are settled, or, if we are unsuccessful after about five days, we will recommend that she come to the in-patient unit. If a person is imminently dying, we will attend daily until death occurs. Since the team has been visiting for a number of days and things are looking better, we are planning to discharge her from our team.

Although frail, Christine is dressed and greets us at the door. I am delighted to see how bright she seems compared with my other visits, but at the same time, I am shocked at how gaunt her face is, and how thin and fragile she has become. She looks so small. We follow her into the living room, where Kelly asks a few questions and then retreats to another room. It's her job to refill the medications and make notes for the home care nurse.

I sit with Christine. I have not spent a lot of time getting to know her, because our visits have focused so much on her physical and spiritual suffering, as she has tried to combine alternative healing with traditional medicine. But today is different. She seems to really want to connect. She shows me pictures of her grown children. She tells me about them, about her life, her dreams. I tell her a bit about my children and my work in Nepal. She recommends a video that I have wanted to see, but have never gotten around to getting a copy. We talk excitedly about it.

"I have a copy; would you like to borrow it?" she says animatedly.

"Really ...?" I say. "I would love to borrow it."

Maybe she senses my hesitation. Is it appropriate to borrow from a patient, I wonder?

"Don't feel that you need to take it—if you're not going to see it ..."

"I want to see it, definitely ..." I assure her. "You'd be doing me a real favour."

When the visit ends, we hug warmly and I wish her well. Kelly has discharged her from our team, so hopefully, I won't see her for a while. As we are driving away, I notice how invigorated I feel. I thank Kelly for giving me space to be with Christine in this way.

"I think that there is a time to engage with people in a casual way, and I really had the feeling today that she wanted to talk ... just about normal things. That's why I engaged with her in a much more personal way than usual," I explain.

"Really?" says Kelly, genuinely interested in my explanation.

"Yeah, I wanted to give her a chance to talk, and to listen, and to still be useful, still contributing. It was kind of sad, though. We were talking about volunteer work and being less materialistic. I felt really sad when she said that she wouldn't need her business clothes anymore. She's going to give them to that organization that provides business clothes for people who can't afford to invest in clothes for the job."

"I got the feeling though, that she knows that her body is changing," says Kelly. "I had a conversation with her partner, Leah. I know she's getting tired, and she was talking a bit about plans for 'after'." Leah has been a devoted caretaker, very loving and attentive to Christine whenever we have been there.

"Yeah," I say. I can really relate to them. "I get it."

My husband and I have some of the same plans to live a simpler life, to travel, and to enjoy our family. Like them, we really enjoy each other's company. And like them, after years as professional healthcare providers, we are preparing to enjoy the rewards of having given a lot to our community. It's just too easy to imagine how disappointing it is for Christine and Leah to be facing each new loss.

I am aware that I am experiencing what is known in the counselling world as counter-transference. I was questioning myself, even as I was talking to Christine in the living room, wondering if our conversation was being helpful to her. Usually, I don't reveal a lot about my own life in conversations with patients and their families, and when I do, I take it as a sign that something is stirring in me, something that may not be of benefit to the patient. On the other hand, identification can be a way to find empathy and compassion and can serve to help me to understand Christine by imagining, in detail, what it would be like to be in her situation. As long as I can keep her experience separate from mine, and keep the focus on her and not me, I can still be of help.

Kelly and I are both silent, left to our own thoughts as I drive us back to the unit. I have a lot of admiration for Christine. She has embraced her illness. Instead of battling or fighting the cancer, she has been trying to understand it and respond to it lovingly through alternative treatments. Her hope has been to coax the cancer to leave her body. She has shown true courage and determination, and despite devastating pain, she has managed to always be welcoming and gracious with our team.

I don't see her again until about four weeks later, on a Sunday afternoon. I come onto the unit and look at the patient board. I say to Kelly, who is on again today, "Christine is on the unit. I think I'll see if I can catch Leah and find out what is happening."

I walk down the corridor and into Room 612, and pause at the door. I see a very small figure in the bed that looks nothing like Christine. I am saddened to see how weak and depleted by the disease she is, and shocked that she looks cachectic—more like a skeleton than a living person. Her breathing has long gaps, her skin is pale and waxy. I pause, trying to take it all in. She is definitely not going to survive this, despite her desire to live. It is hard to witness.

I notice a young man and a young woman sitting on the couch. They must be the children she has told me about. I come a little through the door and introduce myself and ask if I can speak to their mother. They nod, giving permission without words. I kneel by the bedside.

"Christine," I say, "it's Susan. I'm the counsellor who visited you at home. I've come to return your video."

Her eyelids flicker, but she doesn't respond in any other way.

"Christine, the video was good. Thank you."

I take her hand and stroke it. I stay there for what seems like a long time, just matching my breathing to hers. I turn to the adult children, who have been listening to music.

"Can I sit down?" I motion to the couch.

There is something bleak in the way that they are sitting on separate chairs, each lost in their own world of music. When they unplug, I sense awkwardness between them, or maybe it's just that it's hard to believe that they are at hospice, watching their beloved mother dying. They are both on the edge of their chairs.

"Can you tell us what's happening?" says the daughter.

"Yes, I can. It might help though, if I get a nurse to join us. Maybe together we can answer your questions."

"That would be good," the son says, now letting himself relax against the back of the chair.

I go to the charting room, where I can often find the nurse I'm looking for, but the door is shut, which means that they are in rounds and don't want to be disturbed. Then I remember that Kelly is on, and she would be the perfect person to talk to them, as she has visited the house so many times. She comes readily when I ask her. I notice that she slows her pace as she nears the room. Smiling acknowledgement of the adult children, she moves towards Christine. It is affirming to see that her actions mirror mine: she leans in close, taking Christine's hand in one hand, and reaches over with the other to stroke Christine's furrowed brow.

"Christine," she says, "it's Kelly, I'm one of the nurses that visited you at home. Your son and daughter are here, everything is ok."

She stands quietly for some time, continuing to tenderly stroke Christine's forehead, her hair, her face. Her breathing seems to naturally match Christine's. I speak softly to her children, telling them of my wonderful visit.

"I admire your mom so much," I say sincerely.

They respond with weak smiles. Kelly joins us.

"What is your understanding of what's happening?" she asks softly.

They exchange glances. The daughter speaks. "Well, we know where this is going, but ... well is there ... uh anything that can help her? You know ... it's just that ... her breathing ... she's not breathing ... all the time," she says haltingly.

"Yes, that's right ..." says Kelly. "Your mother is going through a natural process. Her body is shutting down, and when that happens, we begin to notice spaces in the breathing." She looks over to Christine, "Like we're seeing right now ... it's a normal part of dying. You've probably noticed that she has gotten sleepier and sleepier. She isn't waking up as much, and she's not had food or water for a few days."

They nod.

"Those are all normal parts of the dying process. She looks peaceful to me."

Silence.

"What do you mean, her body is shutting down?" the daughter asks tentatively, as if she's not sure that she wants to know.

"I see that her heart is working hard, trying to keep the blood going to the vital organs. You'll notice that her fingertips are purplish, or what we call mottled. You'll see the nurses checking her knees and feet. When we see bruising or mottling like she has, we know that death is near. It tells us that the blood flow isn't reaching the periphery."

Kelly pauses for a moment as she takes in their wide-eyed stares.

"Do you want to hear more, or is that enough?" she asks kindly.

They motion for her to continue.

"I'm also noticing that her colour has changed, and that we can hear some fluid accumulating at the back of her throat. You may have heard of the term "death rattle." It can sound like coffee percolating, or like when a kid blows through a straw into a glass of water. If you look carefully, you will see that your mom isn't distressed by it, even though it may sound awful to us. If you have any concerns about it, we can give her medication to dry up the fluid."

They don't say anything, but Kelly and I watch as matching tears slide down their cheeks. Kelly and I don't move, but wait for them to process this information. After a while, the son breaks the silence. "How long," he croaks, "do you think?"

"I don't know for sure, no one knows, but from what we are seeing—her breathing, her sleepiness, her pale skin—I think it could be anytime tonight or maybe in the next few days." Silence.

"Is that what you wanted to know?" I ask.

They both nod.

"It's hard to hear the words spoken isn't it?"

They nod.

"This is your mother."

Silence.

"You really love her."

They nod again, slowly.

We sit in silence. A slight movement perhaps, I'm not sure, but the mood changes. Kelly asks if there is anything else. There is nothing. She leaves, and I offer to make them some tea. When I come back, they are at the bedside, one on either side. They are stroking their mother's face, holding her hands. The sense of them being separate isn't there anymore. They don't seem so awkward.

I sit with them at the foot of the bed and tell them about the video that she lent me, and how inspired I am. I tell them that because their mother gave me that video, I am going to get serious about fundraising so that I can help patients and families in Nepal. The son looks at me. "I gave my mom that video," he says, as a slow smile spreads across his face.

"Really? That's cool."

We continue to talk about his project in a small northern community. He is helping people in isolated communities record the history of their people. He talks passionately about how this gives them dignity and value, and how it preserves their culture. After a while, I say, "I'm going to go now, but I'll check in later, if you like."

The son nods and says, "Yes, that would be good."

It's Thanksgiving—my favourite holiday. It's at Nicole's house. She is my son's girlfriend, and her family has graciously invited our whole family and their partners. They live across the street from the hospital, so it's easy for me to get there. As I walk through the door of their house, I see 15 people squeezed around a dining room table and a kitchen table, pushed together. Every chair in the house is filled with family members, all talking animatedly.

"Mom," my son Malcolm calls out. "Hey, everyone, mom's here."

There are lots of smiles as they make room for me, passing turkey, gravy, mashed potatoes, salads, and vegetables. They are onto dessert and are serving themselves from several big platters. Nicole's dad is filling the wine glasses, but I refuse. "I'm the official driver."

For a half an hour I join in the laughter, eating quickly. The food is good. I think to myself how lucky I am to be able to sit at this table enjoying such good food. Being together is a blessing. I notice that we are not worried, we are not wondering what will happen next. We are taking for granted that everything is fine ... everything is so fine.

I pack up the leftover dessert to share with the nurses who are working on the unit so can't be with their families. I cross the darkened street, the cold wind blowing the glow from my cheeks. Dropping the plate of desserts on the counter in the charting room, I search the board, where our patients' status is noted. I see that Christine has not died while I was out, so I head straight for her room. There sit her son and daughter, each staring into space. It occurs to me that they have not eaten. I ask them.

"Yes," they tell me. "We had breakfast."

I pause, not knowing what to say. "Would you like some pie?"

CHAPTER FIVE:
When resources are lacking counsellors have to make tough decisions

What Validates Our Knowledge?

After returning from a rock-climbing trip, I had an argument with a friend. She was telling the people at a dinner party that she had been very surprised when I had "picked up" a rock climber, who claimed to be a rock-climbing teacher and guide, inviting him to join our group. It came out that she thought that I had been reckless—that I had put my trust in a person about whom I knew nothing—and was risking my life by climbing with him. I was immediately defensive, as her husband began peppering me with questions such as, "What were his credentials?" "Did he belong to an accredited association?" "Who was his teacher?" It had never occurred to me to ask those questions. Even if I had, I wouldn't have known how to evaluate the answers.

To set the context, a brief explanation. When rock climbing, the rope is secured by an *anchor* that the climbers have tied to bolts which they or earlier climbers have embedded into the rock at the top of the rock face. Rock climbing involves at least two people: one who stands at the bottom of the climb and *belays*, or pulls a rope attached to the climber's waist harness, while the other climbs the rock. The action of the belayer tightening the rope prevents the climber from plummeting to the ground, if he or she slips off the rock face.

I thought about our discussion in the days that followed. Had I been rash, even foolish? I had a feeling that I was being unfairly judged, but I didn't know why. I reviewed the scenario. I had met Jack for the first time at the base of the mountain and spent about 30 minutes with him as we hiked to the top of the cliff, while the rest of my group went off in other pairs. After finding a set of bolts to secure our anchor at the top of the climb, Jack tied a selection of knots, demonstrating why one knot might be better than the other, each in different circumstances. As we were solving the problems of building an anchor, he patiently observed my movements, while at the same time providing constructive suggestions.

In retrospect, our earlier conversation, together with his actions (which seemed congruent with my experience of guides and teachers), added up to an authenticity that is difficult to pinpoint, but I nevertheless noticed it and took it in, even if unconsciously. When it came time for both of us to *rappel*—a technique requiring the climber to independently make a controlled descent to the ground—I let him go first. This was my way of ensuring my own safety, because by watching Jack climb down, I was proving that the rope had been tied correctly and would hold our weight. In reviewing the circumstances, I was satisfied that, although I hadn't found out anything about his training or professional affiliations, I *had* made an assessment. I trusted that what he had told me about himself was true, because I trust my own instincts and observation skills. I verified this trust by watching him tie the knots and use the rope, and by allowing him to make the first rappel.

Hold on a minute. This is the concept that I had struggled with in school: epistemology, which has to do with what we believe validates knowledge. Now it made sense! I am a constructivist learner, which means that, for me, learning is a process of constructing with information. And for constructivists, truth is based on social constructs that involve what scholars N.K. Denzin and Y.S. Lincoln (2005) define as "trustworthiness, credibility, transferability, and confirmability" (p.1-33). While one can be objective to a certain degree there is no objective truth. My friends have a different paradigm or model that provides another set of criteria for authenticating what they believe to be true, which explains why they were worried for my safety: I hadn't gone through the steps that they thought would justify my trust in Jack as a partner.

My friends were an airplane pilot and a psychometrician (working with psychological tests), so it is understandable that their training and experience have taught them to rely and depend, primarily, on instruments that provide some objectivity. Writing in *Intuition and Management*, psychiatrist and York University professor Daniel Cappon (1994) says that, "the imperative to follow our own instincts or intuition is so strong that in some professions, people have to be *programmed* to be objective" (p. 22). He gives the example of a pilot "whose every instinct is to trust his own spatial perception, despite the instruments that tell him that he is flying upside down." For people who have been "indoctrinated" in objectivity and have seen for themselves that it is dangerous to trust one's own instincts, it may be hard to understand someone else who has been trained to distrust objective measures, and who puts his or her faith in subjective measures.

Perhaps my friends shared a sense of value, meaning and pride in having overcome obstacles in order to develop an ability to rely on external validation, while I have a sense of value, meaning and pride in having learned to trust my own senses, or internal validation. As well, these primary modes had provided us each with a sense of identity. In his book, *Identity as an Analytic Lens for Research in Education*, researcher and social linguistic scholar James Paul Gee (2000) says that,

> being recognized as a 'kind of person', in a given context" is what forms identity, and the kind of person one is, is recognized as being formed not just from one's core identity—which holds universally for ourselves and others, across contexts—but from "how we perform in society. (p. 99)

He identifies four major contributors to identity: our nature, or the attributes that we carry from birth; our position in society, or our status; our accomplishments; and our affinity groups.

Being a counsellor in a palliative care context both forms and reinforces my identity, by providing me with the opportunity and expectation to enact the "kind of person" that I am—for example, my sensitive nature, my education, my professional expertise, and palliative care values expressed in how I interact with colleagues and families. So, when we attended the home of Mrs. Crosby, as I explain in the next story, I found myself in a position of having to weigh moral, intellectual and emotional criteria to decide on how best to proceed.

Talk About a Job

I'm driving to our next visit, which allows the night nurse, my partner for the evening, to answer the mobile phone. I can only hear Rose's end of the conversation, but I know that she is talking to a home care nurse. Turning to me, she mouths the words: "Hemorrhaging ... Linda Stewart."

"We can't get there," she says into the phone. "Oh dear, it's too late to go to Emergency? I wish we could help, but we have to go to another call. I hope you get there in time. Okay, good luck, and give the family our best ..." She trails off. Hanging up, she turns towards me sadly, shaking her head. "I wish we could get there, but it's just too far." Linda lives near the Red River, which is all the way across town, at least 30 minutes away. "We've already put Mrs. Crosby off. She's been waiting all day."

I'm thinking of Linda and wondering if there will be time to head over there after this visit, but my thoughts are interrupted as the phone rings. Rose fumbles for the mobile in her coat pocket, tensing her body forward in the seat. It's another home care nurse.

"Jason Choo? Yeah, I know who he is. Early thirties, diagnosed three months ago."

'Oh no', I think, 'not Jason'. Jason is a student at the university where I am a student. We had sat in many classes and shared numerous cups of coffee while discussing our upcoming research. I'd heard about his diagnosis. When I recently ran into him, he'd seemed perfectly healthy. Memories interweave with the conversation, and I can only take in snippets as Rose tries to support the nurse on the line.

"Declining rapidly ... terrified ... restless ... mother can't manage ..." The conversation is all moving too fast.

"Okay," I hear Rose say. "I have a visit, and then I have to drive the counsellor home, so I can't get there right away. It will most likely be after midnight. But call me for any reason." She hangs up and looks out the window on her side of the car.

"He's terrified?"

"That's what the home care nurse is saying," she replies, turning to look at me.

Part of me wants to drive right to his house. I could at least comfort his mother. In my imagination I see Jason, reduced to a bare skeleton, his eyes wide, thrashing in his childhood bed.

I flash back to the day that I was the mother, and it was my son lying pale and lifeless on a hospital bed. "No," I mumble out loud. It's too painful to think about. I can't admit to Rose that part of me is relieved that I don't have to go. I'm still thinking about Jason and his mother as we pull up in front of Mrs. Crosby's house. I'm trying to shake it off when I see someone on the porch.

I say, only half-joking, "You know it's going to be a tough visit when the family is waiting on the curb."

We haul out our backpack, briefcase and supply kit, struggling to grab the soaker pads and hospital gowns from the trunk. The man on the front porch ushers us into the house and, without introduction, tells us that his sister has been unable to "piss," adding that she won't stay in bed and keeps falling down when she does get up.

"She's seeing people who aren't there," he says with dismay.

I notice that his face is flushed and his clothes hang limply on his body, except where a small bit of fabric sticks to a wet patch in the centre of his chest. From beneath his faded and stained ball cap, short, greasy clumps of hair stick out at odd angles. We find out that he is Mrs. Crosby's brother, and the woman with her back to us doing dishes is his wife. She occasionally interjects, but her husband is clearly the spokesperson, and he has our full attention as he rapidly fills us in on what has been happening with his sister. There's no pause for us to speak.

After a while, I begin to feel sweaty. Should we be doing something? It's uncomfortable. I am reminded of a slogan posted above the phone in our office, "We are a crisis team, not a team in crisis" and realize that I must attend to my discomfort. I interrupt the flow of Robert's report by asking if I can take a moment to introduce the team.

"Perhaps it would help if I tell you a bit about who we are and what we do," I begin. "We are a 24-hour crisis team. I'm Susan and I'm the counsellor, and this is Rose. She's the nurse," I say, looking over at my partner.

"We're from Meadowview Hospice, and we're known as the Palliative Care Crisis Team, or PCCT. We get called when a registered patient is experiencing symptoms that are not being managed, like pain, restlessness or nausea." I pause, giving them a moment to take it all in. "It was a good decision for you to call. I just want to assure you that we are going to stay here tonight until your sister is settled, or we have another plan in place."

Robert and his wife, who has by now joined us, sit solemnly nodding, but don't respond. I'm not sure what to say.

"We are here to help," I say encouragingly.

Rose takes over and asks them some more questions before focusing on Robert. "Do you think it would be okay if I did a few 'nursie' things—blood pressure, temperature, and feel her tummy?" she asks.

Robert nods his permission.

"Does your sister like to be addressed as Mrs. Crosby, or should I call her by her first name?" Rose asks.

"Betty," says Robert. "Her real name is Elizabeth, but she likes to be called Betty."

His wife leads Rose into the bedroom.

I sense that Robert has something more to say, so I decide to stay with him rather than join Rose. As soon as they leave the room, he pounds his fist on the table and barks out, "The damn doctor! I hate the medical system." His voice grows louder with each statement. "People say it's good here, but they sure haven't done much for my sister."

I wonder if he comes from the United States, but ask, purposely keeping my voice quiet, "What makes you say that?"

"I took her to the doctor, I don't know how many times. He never did any tests. He's just waiting to retire. He doesn't give a flying f."

I say nothing, but keep looking at him.

"And Betty, she didn't want to hurt his feelings. Jeez, can you believe it?"

"That *is* hard to believe," I say, shaking my head.

"I told her. I told her. Oh, what the ... I guess it doesn't matter now ..." His voice trails off, but his eyes remain steady, as if challenging me.

Meeting his gaze with equal intensity, I say, "It must be frustrating to have to wonder if your sister even needs to go through this ... if it could have been prevented."

"Bingo!" he says, half rising from his chair and pointing his finger at my chest. "You got it."

Our conversation is interrupted when Rose enters and pulls up a chair to face Robert, who is seated again.

"I think your sister's condition is changing," she says tenderly, placing her hand on Robert's forearm. "She shouldn't be getting out of bed anymore. She's too weak, and it's not safe."

Robert looks at her somberly as she goes on, tentatively, as if feeling her way. "My understanding is that she wants to die at home." She says it as a statement, but it is a question. "Is that what you and your wife want?"

Robert nods.

"I think the restlessness may be caused by a full bladder, so I'd like to put in a catheter so that she won't have to worry about getting up to the commode."

Robert remains quiet.

"It may help her settle."

Nothing.

"Do you think that would be all right?"

I like the way that Rose is so respectful and sensitive. She can see that Robert is finding it hard to take in what she is saying. Finally, he nods. Noticing that I seem to be connecting with Robert, Rose doesn't ask me to go to the car to get the catheter bag, but instead slips out to get it herself. She returns directly to Betty's bedroom, leaving Robert and I alone to talk.

Robert tells me that he and his wife are caring for two other family members. He says that they can't keep going like this. Betty is the eldest of six siblings, and Robert is the youngest, by 15 years. He and his wife haven't asked for help from anyone, even the other siblings.

"I just feel like it's my duty. When mom died, it was Betty that was there, and now ..." He pauses, lost in thought, then begins again angrily, "I just don't understand how they can justify it—they're too busy? Jeez."

"It's a lot for you to do by yourself," I say.

"It's not that I mind," he sighs, "it's just that, well, it's just the way it is, I guess."

"You've really helped a lot of people, too, and I'm wondering who you turn to when you need help?"

"Oh," he says, giving me a look as if he can't quite make out the meaning of my words. "Well, I have some good buddies ... there's a neighbour. And my son."

"Ah, people who care," I say gently.

"Yeah."

"I wonder if this would be a time when you could turn to them, you know, for some help, ask them to ... even get some groceries, or sit with her while you go for a walk." I let that digest. "You know how much it means to you to help," I say tentatively. "You know, when they see that you are struggling, maybe they don't know how to help. It just might make them feel good, like what you do for Betty," I say haltingly.

"Yeah, it makes you feel better," he says. "To help."

"Yes, it can," I say, "like everyone is in it together. Maybe there are times in life when we have to accept help graciously."

"Your sister seems to be showing you how to do that," I add, as an afterthought.

Rose has quietly re-entered the kitchen and begins counting the syringes to make sure that they have enough medication for the next 24 hours. We hear Betty call out, just before we hear the thump. Rose races to the bedroom and helps Robert's wife get Betty back into bed. I look in a few minutes later, and see Rose stroking Betty's bruised forehead and talking to her quietly. I think to myself that Rose has such a tender heart.

Betty is half-sitting, with one leg out of the bed. She falls back onto the pillows, waving her bony arms in the air. Rose is observing carefully, and I can tell that she is thinking.

"I'm going to have to phone for new orders. She's just not settling," she says decisively, as she glances at her watch. Walking towards the kitchen, she sighs. "I know that your shift is over, and I'm not sure what to do." Rose works until 7:30 in morning, but my shift ends around 11:00 p.m.

"It's okay, Rose, I'll figure it out. It's not your fault. Phone the doctor, and I'll think about it."

She dials the number for one of our regular doctors. "Hi Patty. Mrs. Crosby isn't settling. I've given her two doses, and she's still restless. What do you think? Okay, yup, I'll do that, thank you. Sorry to bother you." She hangs up and looks at me apologetically. "Yeah, I'm going to have to up the medication."

Both of our eyes dart to the filled syringes, neatly lined up by the medication sheet. It will all have to be redone, which can take at least an hour—if Betty settles. If not, it could take longer.

"I just don't feel like I can drive you home, with her so unsettled," Rose continues apologetically.

I don't want her to feel rushed. Robert, who is leaning in the doorway, interjects. "Hey do you need a ride home? I can take you home," he says. "No problem."

I look at Rose. She is nodding. "That's a good idea," she says readily.

I just sit there looking at her, still thinking. I can't phone my boss and ask for overtime, because of the cutbacks, and we're not allowed to call a taxi anymore. There's no use asking for permission anyway, since I'm already late. But it's more than that. I have a really good relationship with my boss. She has told us that the organization is in financial trouble and asked us to be careful about spending. I feel a sense of loyalty to her personally. She wouldn't have asked these things of us if it hadn't been a desperate situation. I don't want to put her in an awkward position, but I feel caught. I have a conviction that the organization should have a realistic sense of the true cost of the program, so I don't want to pay for the taxi myself, or work unpaid overtime. However, I have made a commitment to myself to try to think of the kind and generous thing to do in any given situation. I could ask my husband to pick me up, but he's been painting the house for days, 12 hours up and down ladders. I just don't think it would be fair to disturb him, either.

I'm also thinking about the conversation I've just had with Robert, about accepting help graciously. It occurs to me that, not only would it be hypocritical to refuse his help, it might give us an opportunity to continue our conversation.

"I think that's the best plan," Rose says encouragingly.

"Okay," I say, uncertainly.

Robert leaves Rose and me alone while he goes to get his keys. I turn to Rose and whisper, "Do you think it's unprofessional to accept a ride?"

"No," she says, emphatically, "definitely not."

I'm not sure that she understands my dilemma. I was a child protection worker in the days when treatment for sexual abuse was just being explored. Aside from personal safety issues, I'm thinking about a time when setting appropriate boundaries was the topic of the day. I am known for providing training to counsellors in which I have been adamant about the role of boundaries in protecting the therapeutic relationship. When I came to work at Meadowview, I remember being struck by the way that "appropriate" boundaries were so different in the palliative care world.

For instance, our work at hospice is necessarily intimate. We touch people all the time. Visits usually end with lots of hugs. We are in private spaces—homes, bedrooms, sometimes sitting on the edge of people's beds. Even as a counsellor, I may be called upon to accompany a patient to the toilet, assist the nurse with catheterization, or to look at wounds or open sores. Many bedside conversations are punctuated with retching, vomiting, coughing, leaking, or spewed tears, feces and mucous. My conversations are rarely private. My charting is shared with a variety of other professionals. Boundaries ... I'm just not sure what is appropriate in this situation, but I have agreed to a ride.

I follow Robert to his truck. I can barely step up to the seat, it's so high off the ground. He manoeuvres out of the driveway and very slowly heads down the street, continuing well below the speed limit, which I find puzzling. Feeling the need to fill the silence, I ask him about his work. I am surprised to find out that he makes and collects knives, which he sells on the internet. 'Oh-oh', I think, 'what kind of a man is interested in knives?' Traces of my peace, love and rock and roll days jump to the foreground. A newspaper headline flashes in front of my eyes: "Knife-Lover Kills Unsuspecting ... no, Foolish? ... Counsellor" He flips me a magazine that is lying on the seat between us, featuring a photo of his work on the front cover. It is a photo of three knives that he has crafted. Each one has been made from a different material, and each handle has been hand-carved to look almost lacy. I have to admit that the knives are beautiful, almost delicate in their detail. Each is a work of art. The word "sensitive" comes to mind.

As we head along Sherbrook Street, I notice the huge plane trees along the boulevard, and how the street lights create dappled, flickering shadows in the space between us. Nothing is clear.

"Talk about a job, this must be tough work," he says.

"Believe it or not, I love my job," I respond, almost too enthusiastically.

He half turns in the glowing light of the dashboard. "Really?" he says in surprise, "you actually like it?"

I nod.

"But it must be so sad," he continues incredulously.

"Yes," I agree, "it is sad, even heartbreaking at times, but it's also touching, meeting people." I hesitate. "Like you. It's inspiring. There are so many people who really love other people, who really put out when the going gets tough. It's kind of a privilege, to be part of such an important time ..." Stumbling, not sure what to say next, I add, "If you know what I mean?"

"Yeah," he says, "I guess I do know ... maybe it's like me and Betty ... I was kind of scared when she first got sick, but it really hasn't been so bad. We've become close in a way that we hadn't been before."

"Yes," I say, "when we care for someone, do the physical care, we don't feel so helpless, and I think that maybe if we are not protected from it, and we're able to be right there, you know ... as our elders go through the process, dying really does become a part of life, and when it comes to be our time ... well, it's not so unknown, not so scary ... "

As we arrive at my street, I wonder if I should reveal to him where my house is, but it would seem too awkward, even offensive, to ask to get off at the corner, so I point to my house. As I open the door of the truck, he says, "Look, Susan, I ... um ... want to thank you for your help tonight," his voice catching. "It really makes a difference."

"Thank you. And thanks for the ride too, you really helped me out." I notice that he waits until I am inside the door before driving away.

The next day, I'm sitting in the community office when one of the nurses, who helps us when the team is busy, walks in. Dropping her bags on the floor, she falls into the chair at the table. We chat amiably before I ask her if she has heard about what happened with Jason last night.

"Yeah," she says sadly, "he died before Rose could get there. She was pretty broken up about it."

I feel badly for Jason and his mom. I feel badly for Rose. One of the strengths and weaknesses of nurses on our team is that they take their responsibilities very seriously, and I know that for Rose, not being able to help someone in need will be really hard for her. Rose has a huge heart. Sometimes, no matter how much we do, it's still not enough. I blink back tears.

"Sometimes it's just so sad," Wanda empathizes.

After a moment I ask, "Linda Stewart?"

"I heard that she died quickly. Her family was okay."

There is a pause as we each retreat into our own thoughts. Breaking the silence, Wanda asks if I want to hear about her visit with Betty this morning.

"Yes, of course." I lean forward eagerly.

"Robert told me how much he appreciated your visit last night. He said he got a lot out of his conversation with you ... about how it's okay to accept help, and all that you said about the natural process of dying. He really liked the part about how helping his sister helps him to prepare for his own death."

I smile at her. "Thanks Wanda. Thanks for letting me know, it really means a lot to me." I reach out and give her a big hug.

CHAPTER SIX:
Everyone on the team needs emotional support

Dinner and Stories

Although a counsellor's main role is to serve patients and families, we also have responsibility for supporting the psychological well-being of the entire team. We often design and deliver workshops that help staff deal with difficult issues, such as providing spiritual care, dealing with conflict, or self-care. My doctoral research revealed that creative processes could provide a safe space to bear witness, to connect with others, and to explore difficult events.

So, with this in mind, I created what I called "Dinner and Stories": I invited people from all areas of our hospice organization—housekeepers, managers, supervisors, front desk clerks, nurses, doctors, volunteers, counsellors and fundraisers—to come in small groups to my house, where I created a safe space for us to share some of our experiences. I began with participants sharing "something wonderful," with the group. This could be absolutely anything—an object, a photo, a poem, a song. I intentionally left the instructions vague, so that people could use their imaginations. When participants arrived, I served appetizers and tea and gave each person a chance to share what they had brought. This helped to ease any tension, since many of the participants did not know each other well, if at all.

Then we broke for a dinner that I had designed with the particular participants in mind: I catered to likes and dislikes, which I had asked them to communicate to me by email, to confirm their attendance and food preferences. I served the dinners with wine, and there was lots of interesting conversation unrelated to work, as well as a good serving of hilarity. After dessert, I poured more tea, and we moved back into the living room to read stories. Again, to lighten any tension and normalize performance anxiety, I told the story about a writing group I had been in where we had discovered the value of a "group apology." In this apology, everyone speaks at once and "apologizes" for their writing being ... too short, too long, not creative, badly written, not that interesting. This usually ends in hearty laughter.

Another benefit of the group is that, as the group leader, I can model vulnerability and also self-reflection. On the first of these evenings, after the group apology, when it was my turn, I read a story about a visit in which the crisis team was called to the home of a young woman. I had not shared this story with anyone, other than in a brief chat with my supervisor at the time it happened. This is the story that I read.

The Medic's Daughter

It was towards the end of my shift, when we were called out to the home of a young woman, technically an adult but still living with her parents. Counsellors work either from 7:00 a.m. to 3:00 p.m. or 3:00 p.m. until 11:00 p.m. Nurses work 12-hour shifts, from 7:30 to 7:30. Although my shift was officially coming to an end, and the nurse would normally have continued until 7:30 a.m. alone, I went with her, because our team had agreed that nurses should not attend the death of a child or a young person by themselves.

When we entered the home, the family dispersed as we introduced ourselves to the young woman's father. We were ushered to the family room, where the girl's body lay. The family members did not make eye contact with me, even when I introduced myself. Neither did they respond to my questions and comments. I interpreted this to mean that they did not want to engage with me, or, more specifically, with a counsellor. The father, who was a medic in the military, directed all comments to the nurse.

I could hear activity in the background, and I had the sense of frantic, urgent energy in the house. The nurse had experience as a medic and, as she told me later, she had noticed the father's rather strange way of relating and had made a conscious decision to speak his "lingo" as a way of developing rapport. They spoke rapidly, and I found the conversation hard to follow, partially because it was late and I was tired, and partially because they were using abbreviations and jargon that I didn't understand to do with arranging ambulance transport. I didn't think it was appropriate to clarify, so I stood back a bit, trying as best I could to make sense of what they were saying.

The father indicated to the nurse that he wanted his daughter's body removed as soon as possible, but unfortunately, there had been a huge accident on the highway, and all of the transport vehicles were busy. My partner put some calls in to the dispatchers, but they were not returning her messages. We sat awkwardly with some family members, around the young woman's body, which was laid out on her bed. Both the nurse and I tried to engage the family in conversation, but they clearly were not interested. The father, pointing to the daughter, was saying things like, "That's not my daughter," and "We have to get that thing out of here." Then the mother and sister started making jokes about the way she looked. To my horror, they got out some face paint and drew a clown's face on her, then began pinching her lips to make it seem like she was talking, followed by lifting her arms up and waving them in the air, as if she was punctuating her comments with gestures.

I sat in stunned silence, not knowing how to respond. When the phone rang, the nurse took the call, removing herself from the scene. I could hear her trying to advocate for transport to come as soon as possible. The father kept coming and going from the room, and at one point I could hear him in the hallway, speaking in a loud voice to someone else. The nurse went to talk to him when she got off the phone, and I heard him making demands, and with a raised voice insisting that, "If someone doesn't come and get that thing out of here in the next 10 minutes, I swear I'll roll it up in a blanket and transport it myself!"

I had no doubt that he would do exactly that. The nurse came back and gave me a look of helplessness as she dialled the phone and spoke adamantly to the dispatcher, once again. I remained by myself, sitting next to the girl's body, feeling useless. The girl's cousin came and sat beside me. She seemed like she had something to say, but when I tried to engage her in conversation, she became remote, and then got up and drifted into another room. Later, the nurse told me that she had looked over and thought I looked forlorn. That word stayed with me, because it described exactly what I was feeling. I was forlorn.

After a very long and strained wait, transport was arranged, and we left. On the way home, the nurse and I had an animated discussion about what happened. I had a sincere desire to understand this family's behaviour. I was trying to imagine what would have to happen that would allow me to refer to my beloved child's body as "that thing." I was thinking of my son's death when he was a baby, and I described to the nurse how beautiful his body was after he died ... his pale, translucent skin, his tiny fingers, and how I had held him and kissed him and tried to take in his smell. I remembered looking at his eyelids and thinking that it was so sad that they would never open again. I had behaved so differently from these family members. Was it because Dante was just a baby when he died? I then tried to imagine my adult son lying dead in our family room, and I made myself imagine laughing and making fun of him, but the thought was just horrible.

The nurse and I then started talking about where we had gotten the idea that a body must be treated with respect. Did this behaviour help the family to distance from their grief? Why do we treat the body with respect?

"Ok," I said, "the body houses the spirit, and once the spirit is gone the 'person' isn't there anymore. I remember my Catholic friend in high school telling me, in a mocking tone, that the body is a temple for the soul and should be treated that way. I think she was making fun of the idea, because it had something to do with refraining from sex, but that phrase has stayed with me, and I think it is a lovely way to think of the body. How do we make the transition from caring for this sacred temple, to then burning or burying the temple? I think that, culturally, we have been taught to have respect for the body as a way to bridge making cremation or burial meaningful."

What was happening for these people? I couldn't figure it out, but neither could I shake the feeling that I had witnessed something that was "just wrong." I had the feeling that I might have had if I were to have witnessed racism or bullying and not done or said anything, like somehow, I had become a party to it. I felt bereft that I could not have found some inroad into this family, some way that I could have helped them. What could I have done or said? Although I did speak about this incident with my supervisor, I felt protective of him, because I knew that he knew the family socially, and I didn't want him to think badly of them.

Now I am left with the ghastly image of what I believe was a desecration of a body, and I wonder if the family looks back with shame on their actions, and if they do, can they forgive themselves? They were in shock, and I believe that they were doing the best they could to try to integrate this horrendous loss. I hope that they found solace in knowing that they had cared for her.

The first time that I read this story to my colleagues, I was overcome by their warmth, heartened that they, too, found the situation difficult, and that they agreed they wouldn't have known what to do either. It was affirming to see that my colleagues were moved, and very forgiving of me. But it seems that I wasn't finished with the story.

Here is what I wrote to my colleagues who attended the first and second dinners.

Dear Colleagues,

I have been thinking about the story I wrote about a situation where a family had struggled with their daughter's body remaining in the home. For those of you who were at the dinner when I first read the story, you may remember that I was tearful when I remembered my own son's body after he died, and later when I described what I thought was bizarre behaviour on the part of the family towards the girl's body. I felt better after reading my story, and I appreciated the discussion.

As the time neared for the second dinner, I wrote another story, but at the last minute decided that I wanted to read "The Medic's Daughter" again. This time, as those of you who were there could clearly see, I was overcome with emotion, and at several points could barely get the words out. As happened in the first group, I felt cared for, and I gained new insight from the discussion. I thought that surely, I was "finished" with that story. But no, there was more.

Why did I have so much feeling about the events that had taken place, and why did it seem to grow rather than diminish after telling it the second time? Was there something missing? I decided that the story needed a different ending, or perhaps there is no real ending, but rather a re/visioning.

My original apology still stands, so I need not repeat it here. Actually, on second thought—no apology needed.

Upon reflection, I realized that there was a reason I had not discussed this incident or my feelings with the nurse I had been with, other than in the car on the way home, or with anyone else after I spoke to my supervisor the day after it happened. I realized that I have felt ashamed. I did not want to reveal what I thought of as my inadequacy. Paradoxically, after telling the story twice, rather than feeling inadequate and diminished, as I had feared, I feel almost exhilarated, freed from the prison of "not enough," a feeling that has dogged me throughout my life. At this moment, I see myself not through the eyes of my critic who is never satisfied, who rails at my passivity and is scathing of my seemingly unending need to express my feelings. Instead, I see myself as reflected through your eyes, and in so doing, I feel completely adequate. At least for today, for this moment, I am enough! What a beautiful feeling. Aside from my "role" as a counsellor and colleague, more importantly, I am a person. I am a person who is perfectly living out what it means to be human, and my story is my way of letting you see the person that I am, beyond the role. I see that you see me!

Here it is again:

What was happening for these people? I couldn't figure it out, but neither could I shake the feeling that I had witnessed something that was "just wrong." I had the feeling that I might have had if I were to have witnessed racism or bullying and not done or said anything, like somehow, I had become a party to it. I felt bereft that I could not have found some inroad into this family, some way that I could have helped them. What could I have done or said? Although I did speak about this incident with my supervisor, I felt protective of him, because I knew that he knew the family socially, and I didn't want him to think badly of them.

Now I am left with the ghastly image of what I believe was a desecration of a body, and I wonder if the family looks back with shame on their actions, and if they do, can they forgive themselves? They were in shock, and I believe that they were doing the best they could to try to integrate this horrendous loss. I hope that they found solace in knowing that they had cared for her.

Today, as I hold the nurse, the family, the young woman and myself in my imagination, my future self—future-Susan—goes back into that room. She stands in the corner and beholds the nurse putting aside her own feelings of horror at the family's behaviour, harnessing her ability to navigate a complicated bureaucratic structure to get help for a family that is barking orders at her, with no help from her colleague.

Future-Susan sees a family that has been forced to bear witness to the suffering of their most precious loved one, a family who has tenderly cared for her and simply cannot make sense of this body that lays on the bed, this body that bears a macabre resemblance to the living, breathing person who once was, but who has now become a symbol of their complete failure to stop their beloved from being annihilated, wiped out, gone ... forever.

Future-Susan sees the young woman's body and imagines her spirit: a strong spirit that had a whole life that might have been. She imagines this being battling with all the energy and will of a young person, her soul fighting to endure, to stay and live the life that she felt entitled to, not just for herself, but to ease the suffering that she could plainly see as her parents, sister and friends supported her. The last thing she would have wanted was to cause them pain.

Future-Susan sees past-Susan sitting forlornly—alone, and in despair. Future-Susan moves from the corner where she has been quietly watching and stands firmly behind the nurse, embracing and gently rocking that part of the nurse that has been denied, rudely shoved aside, simply trying to do her job. Future-Susan whispers, "You are valuable, you are safe."

She gathers each family member, and takes all of them together into her arms. She holds them and kisses them on their cheeks and whispers, "You are loved."

Future-Susan kneels beside the girl's bed and bows to the temple lying there, and silently, tenderly says, "You are beautiful." Taking past-Susan into her arms, and next to her heart, she strokes her hair and whispers in her ear, "Do not despair, for you are not alone." She says this because future-Susan knows that someday, past-Susan will find the right time, the right place, and the right people and she will tell her story and be held with this same tenderness.

When that day comes, past-Susan does tell her story, and her colleagues listen, and through their compassion, she does come to know that she is not alone. When she tells her story, her medical colleagues understand that sometimes, there are situations that their counselling colleagues find so overwhelming that they are not able to overcome them in the moment. On behalf of *the* nurse in this story, they will forgive past-Susan for not knowing how to help the nurse.

Her counselling colleagues will understand that when feelings are overwhelming, it is impossible to be effective in the way that she had intended; in the way that she had hoped and wanted to be. When she tells her story, the counsellors will forgive *the* counsellor in this story for dissociating when things got to be too much. They will forgive *the* counsellor for being unable to use her training and her skills to penetrate the barriers that were meant to protect the family from harm, but also prevented them from feeling loved. They will forgive *the* counsellor in the story for carrying unending, sometimes paralyzing grief that makes it impossible to connect with other people.

Those in her group who are parents, sisters, brothers and friends will allow themselves to feel, just for a moment, the tremendous loss of a child and will forgive *the* family members in this story for behaviour that seems so incomprehensible. Her colleagues whose role it is to communicate to the public about hospice, and to raise funds, and those who are doctors, nurses and counsellors and also help to create an image of hospice being a caring refuge, will recognize that there is and always will be an underside to who we seem to be. There is a cost to excellent, compassionate care that cannot be measured in dollars. They will realize that there is an exchange that takes place, and it is only beneficial to all—that is, it will only work if patients and families *and*, not *or*, caregivers have a safe and supportive space in which to grow from their experiences, and where we, as professional caregivers, can fully explore our own humanity. Perhaps they will keep this in mind when securing funds.

The people in the groups with whom she has shared her story will be with past-Susan and with future-Susan, in the room with their nursing colleague, in the room where the medic's daughter lies with her family around her. They will, at least for this moment, accept the complete nakedness of these human beings who are vulnerable because they love. They will, even if only for a moment, join the company of all human beings who have loved and been hurt ... with all human beings who have ever felt that they were not enough. They will feel hope. They may even hear the distant voice of their own future selves, whispering with compassion and love: "You are valuable." "You are safe." "You are loved." "You are beautiful." "You are not alone."

And finally, they may know, if only for a moment, that they too are enough.

CHAPTER SEVEN:
Not living up to our own standards is painful

Whenever People are Involved, it is Complex

Although many counsellors arrived at their jobs at hospice following an event that involved loss, counsellor's lives of course do not remain static. It is not as if we have dealt with grief, and now we can serve others. No. Our lives continue to unfold, and we have high expectations of ourselves when it comes to our own families. But finding compassion for patients and their families and being intimate is different at work than it is in our personal lives. In palliative care encounters, we meet because of our roles.

In his book, *Relational Being*, psychologist and professor at Swarthmore College, Kenneth Gergen (2009), observed that virtually all intelligible action is born, sustained, and/or extinguished within the ongoing process of relationship. From this standpoint, there is no isolated self or fully private experience. Rather, we exist in a world of co-constitution. We are always already emerging from relationship; we cannot step out of relationship; even in our most private moments, we are never alone.

I am a social constructivist, so I see it from this point of view: the players are both given the opportunity to meet because of the context of palliative care, and they are limited by the social expectations of the roles that they inevitably play. For instance, a "counsellor" is expected to interact in particular ways that have been pre-defined and are at least, to some extent, understood. The same can be said for the role of "nurse," "patient," or "family member."

Palliative care values require us to transcend our professional roles in order to connect as human beings. All of the players will, however, always be in flux between our being-ness and the world. In other words, in the palliative care context, I will always be moving between interacting with the other in my role as a counsellor, and interacting with the other as a human being encountering mortality. In this context, then, the other can also move between interacting with me in his or her role as the patient, and interacting with me in his or her role as a human being encountering mortality. It is not that we cannot or are not enacting our humanness, but more that the role to some extent defines, controls and contains what is expressed and what is censored.

In the palliative care literature, it is sometimes written that professionals who do "emotional labour" are "performing" compassion when we work with patients and families, implying that we have the ability to summon feelings "as if" an event was happening to our own mother, child or spouse. My feeling of what it might be like "if" my husband was dying is not the same as what I would feel were he actually dying. Of course! How else could it be? When I recently got the news that a friend has prostate cancer, I immediately thought of all the social situations we had shared, and especially about his quirky sense of humour. Then I flashed forward to holidays, dinners and afternoon walks without him, and the picture seemed so empty and flat without his presence. Our plans to travel just will not happen without him. Then I imagined supporting his wife, possibly for years, as she goes through the painful adjustment to being single again. My response was a complicated ball of emotion that cannot be isolated from my past or my future. I do not have that past or future with the patients and families I visit during my work day.

Perhaps it is as Danai Papadatou (2009) said, that when we are in a professional role, we practise holding both our own perspective and our imaginative idea of what another's perspective might be. To perform can mean to act, say by simulating or feigning an emotion, or behaving in a way that suggests a particular emotion, quality or characteristic. Are we merely simulating emotion? Are we displaying mannerisms that are suggestive of the real thing, the real emotion, or the real caring person? To perform can also mean to carry out, or accomplish something up to an expected standard. Might that imply that we are simply carrying out the "job" of compassion? It does not feel like that to me. There seems to be some truth in how we respond to grief in the standard or expected way—with caring, with compassion, with kindness—while each giving something of ourselves that is unique and what I would call precious, which "standard," or "expected" does not encapsulate.

My colleagues agree with me that the feelings that arise when we connect with families and patients are genuinely compassionate. But our interactions have neither the depth nor the complex set of ties that take years to develop. Imagination is not the real thing, as anyone who has ever had a person close to them die will tell you. Although we can be empathetic by drawing on real feelings, we cannot be expected to share the depth or breadth of grief of the people whose lives are being directly affected.

However, whenever people are involved, it is complex. Shortly after I came to work at hospice, my mother came to live with my family. I had no real idea of what dementia was, although I had seen some patients who were confused. I hadn't really taken in what that might mean to the family, and I did not hesitate to be there for my mom because, well, she needed me. This was consistent with who I believed I was. But the following story illustrates that who I want to be is not necessarily who I am.

A Fate Worse Than Death

My identity is as an empathetic person: I take care of people. It's my job. I'm an expert in grief and loss, in more ways than one, so it's not easy to remember a time when I didn't know what grief looked and felt like. My work as a counsellor has centred on supporting the dying and those who grieve, which makes it difficult to admit that I was unable to give that same support to my mother in the years leading up to her diagnosis of Alzheimer's disease. I wanted to be a loving person, I wanted to care for her, I wanted to be a role model for my children. I wanted to do what I thought—and still think is—just the right thing to do.

It was only towards the end, as I was ready to put her in the dreaded old folk's home, when someone handed me an article on dementia and grief in caregivers, that I really got it that my mother was dying, albeit very slowly, and that I was grieving the loss of her, day by day. Up until that time, no one actually told me that a diagnosis of Alzheimer's disease or dementia is a palliative diagnosis, although one might wonder why I didn't know that. I didn't know then that what I was about to experience—love and goodwill that slowly dissolved into impatience, intolerance, irritation and finally, rage and hatred— was common to other caregivers, and that my confusion and shame about my emotional response was mixed up with my grief.

I've always had a strong sense of family values, and I wanted my children to grow up learning by example that part of being in a family, in a community, means that we help each other. I told my mom that there would always be a place for her at my house, and that I would consider it an honour if she were to live with me. Her own father had been "shared" among her siblings, and I remembered, as a child, the joy when it was our "turn" to have him stay with us. My mother certainly considered it an honour to care for her father. So, what happened?

Mom was a typical woman of her time, and like many women of the 1950s, she had dedicated herself to our home and family, catered to my dad, took delight in her kids and loved shopping at the mall. She had a few aspects to her personality that I didn't particularly like ... the tendency to gossip, fearfulness, insecurity, and a continual need for reassurance. These were just aspects of her personality that I was aware of, wished were different, but accepted.

Before the sudden death of my dad in 1984, she was fun, adventurous, always up for a good time, ready to comfort, and willing to pitch in and help. After dad died, Mom leaned heavily on my brother for emotional support, while at the same time, he stepped to the helm of the family business. My mom's sister came to stay with her for a month to help her out, but one day when she didn't come out of her bedroom, my mom knocked on the door, and when there was no answer, walked in to find that she had died from a heart attack. My brother accompanied the body and my mom back to the United States for the funeral. We all agreed, "poor mom," and our hearts went out to her.

But it got worse. A few months later, my brother was washing the dishes, complained about a headache and asked his wife to call an ambulance. His last words were, "I don't think I'm going to make it." He had an undiagnosed and rare form of leukemia, and he died before he got to the hospital. We were all in shock. I had given birth to my second child during this period, and my sisters had small children, as well. Some of us were also working or going to school. It wasn't surprising when my mom showed an inability to function, or when she couldn't make the simplest of decisions. My sisters and I, overcome by our own grief, tried to manage our responsibilities, small children, jobs and school, while at the same time helping mom adjust. But mom's grief seemed to get worse. Her insecurity became overwhelming and debilitating, and the more we did, the more critical she became, and the more helpless she was in being able to do for herself. On top of all this, our family business had to be run, so my eldest sister jumped in to try to save the family fortune.

The stress of all of this continued for several years, and our family relations deteriorated as we struggled to get through our own grief, attend to our small children and manage the business that my brother had been groomed to take over and which now had no manager. There was family dissent, and we ended up in bitter fights and a lawsuit with my sister-in-law. We fanned out, staying in our corners, licking our wounds.

My mother was in contact with all of my sisters, and she began reporting nasty stories about one sister or another. At that point, it never occurred to anyone to speak directly with each other. Whatever thoughts we had about each other, we kept to ourselves or in private conversations with our spouses, but each of us, for our own reasons, felt growing resentment, which began to include my mother. One day, in a rare visit with my eldest sister, I blurted out, "You know, I'm not sure I really like mom anymore." It was a shocking statement.

My niece, who needed a place to stay, agreed to move in with mom to help her out. But before long, the stories my mom told about her were so disturbing that we began to worry about what was going on over there, until gradually the stories became so ridiculous that we knew something was not right. Mom complained that her granddaughter invited her out to dinner but "forgot" her wallet, or kept the house messy, or other minor complaints. When we talked with my niece, she told a different story: how she had tried to talk about mom's complaints, and how mom had told her not to worry about these things. This version made more sense to us than my mother's version. Then my mom's complaints became ridiculous, such as bitterly reporting that my niece had eaten a "whole" orange, or that she had turned the radio on, or that she had done two loads of laundry. We didn't know what to make of all this, because it seemed like more of the gossip to which we had been accustomed.

One day, my mom made a frantic phone call to my sister. She was crying so hard that she was unable to speak. When she finally settled down enough to get words out, she said that she couldn't figure out what time it was. She haltingly explained that she had gone out on the street to ask people what time it was, and each person said something different ... 12 o'clock, 10 to 12, around 12. "What am I supposed to do?" she sobbed. My sister was silent, not being sure how to respond, but eventually she told her to look at the digital clock by her bed and read her the numbers.

"12: 30," my mom read.

"Okay, that's the time," my sister said.

Susan Breiddal

"Oh. Is that how you do it? Just read the numbers?"

"Yes, that's how you do it," my sister said.

"Oh, no one ever told me that."

Dementia had happened so gradually that we hadn't recognized it.

Since mom refused to see a doctor, we phoned his office and asked the receptionist to call mom and tell her that the doctor wanted to see her. Being old school, my mom didn't question the request. When she came home, my sister asked her what he had to say and she said, "Dementia! I don't like that word."

We didn't like it either, but we didn't really know what it meant. We were about to find out.

After a number of stories my mom told with great humour about being lost—ending with one in which she was going down the highway on the wrong side of the road, and in her attempt to turn the car around got stuck on the median—my sisters and I made the difficult decision to take away her car keys. We tried to talk about it with her, reasoning that she would be very upset if she hurt someone, but she was having none of it. "Everyone gets lost from time to time," she said indignantly.

After a while, my sister asked to borrow her car while her own was getting fixed. My mom agreed, and my sister took the keys and the car. Later, my mother phoned me to report that my sister had taken the car and wouldn't give it back. Up until that time, stories such as this had been told without challenge. We hadn't phoned our siblings and said,

132

"So what's happening, mom says you took her car and won't give it back?" That would have been so simple, but we really hadn't thought about intervening. We might have just thought that that particular sibling was taking advantage and been somewhat angry. But now we knew that we would have to meet and talk about everything. This was difficult, given that bad relations had developed, at least in part, by the patterns of indirect communication that was our main mode at the time.

The stress was enormous for my eldest sister. She went into my dad's office every day and sat at his desk, surrounded by his papers, as she tried to finish a huge job for which the company was responsible. Her only preparation for running a construction company was having worked in the office when she was a teenager. At the same time, she had the task of shutting down the company. She left her job as an art teacher and did her best to wind up a $4-million construction job and a $2-million company. The combination of extreme stress, grief, and previously poor communication habits brought our family to its knees. We could barely speak to each other.

Throughout this time, my mom seemed to have no awareness that my sisters and I were deeply grieving, having lost a father, aunt and brother. She seemed oblivious to what we might need, almost as if she was paralyzed, and she relied on my sister for everything: from going through the huge family home and boxing up everything, to selling it,

choosing and arranging for finances to buy a con-
dominium, moving, refurnishing, and redecorating.
I remember being at her condo once, and overhear-
ing a conversation with my sister. It was 7:00 a.m.,
and mom had tearfully phoned her because she
couldn't decide which colour curtains she should
order. My sister, who was getting three children
ready for school and daycare and trying to get to
work on time, promised to come over before dinner
to help her choose the fabric.

When it finally became clear to us that mom was
no longer able to function on her own, my sisters
and I met to decide what to do. One of our main
dilemmas was trying to determine how much right
we had to interfere in her life. She had fairly easily
agreed for us to take over the finances when we suggested that she had earned the right to be relieved of
that duty. But we wondered if it was okay to phone
her doctor and let him know that she wasn't doing
well. Was it okay to set up a taxi account that was
paid for with her money (which we knew she would
never agree to), telling her, instead, that it would be
paid for by the company, something that dad would
have wanted her to have? Was it okay to make plans
for her without her input? We knew that we had
to act. My eldest sister was the spokesperson, and
she tried to gently suggest that it might be time for
her to move to a place where she could get a bit of
help. This was met with outrage. My mother was,
and always had been, dead set against anything that

was connected to the elderly, and she couldn't say the word "seniors" without disgust and contempt. She did not want to be "lumped together with old people."

After another tearful phone call, this time about not knowing how to turn on the taps, she finally agreed to move in with me and my family, whom she came to refer to as "the Victoria people" when she phoned my sisters to report.

"Those Victoria people ..." she would say, "they're not very nice, they wake me up in the middle of the night and ask me if I want dinner," referring to times when we woke her after she fell asleep in front of the TV in the afternoon. "I know exactly what they're up to."

"What, mom?" my sisters would ask, with concern in their voices. "What are the Victoria people up to?"

"Trying to make me look stupid."

We put her name on a wait list for a facility—not that we wanted to put her in one, but simply to have the choice, as we had heard that the wait lists were long. My youngest sister and I went to look at a few of the places, and we were absolutely appalled. We could not imagine our mother in a place that had elderly people lined up in wheelchairs in the hall, chins on chests, the institutional smell barely masking the smell of urine, feces, and what seemed like rotting flesh. We vowed that we would never do such a thing to our mother. As it turned out, in the two and a half years that she was on the wait-list, we were continually told that it would be another six months. Her name did not move up on the list by even one spot.

However, life with my mom was becoming extremely difficult. The social worker told me to think of the nasty comments, the racist remarks spoken loudly in public, the physical attacks on my young son for no apparent reason, as not really being my mother. That's a common piece of advice. The problem was that some of it—the gossip and the nasty comments to third parties—was just like my mother, but it was as if the part of her brain that has been socialized or provided a censor dissolved, and her anxiety and pettiness was a hundred times magnified.

Why couldn't her sense of humour and childlike delight have become magnified? Not that there weren't humorous moments. One night, while watching an old Christmas special on television, she made a comment about the host, who had died several years before. "I know that he's dead, and I can understand how they make his arms and legs move ... but what I don't get is ... *how* did they get his lips to move?"

We were adaptable and creative. We hired students to introduce themselves as friends, since she claimed that she didn't need any help. They took her shopping, sightseeing, and out to lunch. Things were manageable, until the point where she was unable to dress herself and unwilling to brush her teeth or take a bath. I didn't know what to do. She wouldn't allow us to help her, because they "didn't do those things in my day." She had lost her sense of smell as a young child and had always asked us to be honest with her about whether or not she smelled. When I gently reminded her that she had told me to tell her if she ever smelled badly, and said that it seemed like she may need to change her underwear, she looked at me in horror, her eyes squinting with hatred, and told me that she promised herself she would never let herself be treated so rudely. She refused to take a bath. I didn't know then that people with dementia can lose their depth perception and have the sense that they are getting into a deep pool with no bottom, which is why they avoid the bath.

She was anxious. She spent her days in endless pursuit of her purse or her comb, unable to rest until they were found, but immediately misplacing them, only to frantically and tearfully start looking for them again. She became impatient with the children, accusing them of changing the channels or taking the biggest piece of cake, or, one day, walking up behind my eight-year-old son and giving him a strong punch, saying, "How do you like that?" One day, she turned around in a movie theatre and hit a young girl with her purse because she was kicking the back of her chair. When my 11-year-old daughter said, "Gram, it isn't nice to hit people," she giggled and said, "I know ... but I just wanted to."

I was torn by loyalty to my family and a sense of duty to my mom, so I was dismayed and deeply disappointed in myself as I realized that I was feeling more than mild dislike for my mother. What was happening to me? I had always thought of myself as kind and loving, and capable of facing adversity, especially on an emotional level. Where was the loving part, the patient part, the part that would do anything for my mother? What about being a good model for my kids? Not only could I not care for her, I hated her. I cried at night, asking God to melt my hatred and replace it with love. I had this idea that later, I would look back and know what I should have done. But I wanted to know now, while I could still make things right. "Please God, help me to know now," I would cry in despair.

"I'm doing my best," I would say defensively to my husband. But what if your best isn't enough? What if I *wasn't* doing my best? I would resolve to try harder to be patient. But when my husband, who had been extremely kind and loving, told me that he was feeling depressed, I finally, with the support of my sisters, made the heartbreaking decision to put mom in a facility.

We had her name on the list for a bed in Victoria for two and a half years, but because of a shortage, she had not moved any closer to the top of the list. We were told that we could take her to Emergency and leave her there, and that she would be put in a "holding" place in the psychiatric ward until a bed came free. I just couldn't do that, knowing how frightened and disoriented she would be. So, we decided to move her back to Vancouver and take the first bed we could get, which was way out of town, making it very difficult for my sisters and me to visit.

When I told my mother that she would be going to a place in Vancouver, she was furious and said that she would run away. Because she couldn't remember, we had this conversation several times, each time as if it was the first. Finally, I wrote a note and put it on the table. Every time she read the note, she became angry. One time, she said she was so angry that she wanted to throw the salt and pepper shakers at me. When the day came for her to move, I drove the car with her things, and a kind friend took her home and laced her coffee with lorazepam (usually used to treat anxiety), to try to prevent her from jumping out of the van, as she had done once before.

Words cannot possibly describe the despair I felt when I got to the "home" and saw the empty, lifeless halls. No one greeted us. No one offered support. We found a care aide who gave us the room number, and we put her pictures on the wall and made up her bed. I am left with a haunting memory of my mom standing in the hall looking small, frail and completely lost, and I am reminded of the inscription from Dante as he passes through the gates of Hell in the *Inferno*: "Abandon hope, all ye who enter here."

You may have heard the phrase "a fate worse than death." After my dad, aunt and brother had died, I had faced another series of deaths, including that of my infant son, followed by both of my husband's parents. Understandably, I thought that death was the worst thing that could happen. Over the time my mother lived with us, I found out that there is a fate worse than death: I think it is worse to find that you are alienated from a family you once loved and were loved by. I think it is worse to live with the stress of not understanding anything around you, being with "strangers" who may or may not have ill wishes for you, of having a sense that you are supposed to be doing something or going somewhere, and that you will be in trouble if you don't get there or do it immediately—but you have no idea what that is. And if this goes on indefinitely, it becomes a living nightmare. For instance, mom told me that her boyfriend had taken her to a movie. I asked her what she meant, and she said that John had taken her to a movie. I tried to be helpful and said, "Oh mom, John isn't your boyfriend, he's Lynda's husband."

"What?" she said, clearly shocked at this stunning betrayal. "Lynda married my boyfriend?"

It is indeed a fate worse than death to believe that the people who are trying to help you are out to hurt you, or that the care aides are trying to sexually abuse you, or that your family is going to put you out onto the street or is trying to trick you in some way.

It wouldn't be accurate to say that there was nothing I could do for her. I did provide a home in the community for her for several years. I hired loving people to spend time with her. I cooked great meals. My husband and my kids were patient and loving, and mom was included in all family events. So why do I feel guilty? I cannot completely forgive myself for not being able to love her. I know now that I was angry because the mother I knew was disappearing before my eyes, and somehow, I thought that she had control but was choosing not to use it. I know that I was angry, because I couldn't find the love and patience that I saw others demonstrating, and that I felt and acted upon in my own work. I felt deep shame for being so unloving—whether it showed or not, and whether or not other people think that I tried. *I know* that I hated her.

There were two things that I needed more than anything else. The first was accurate and complete information about dementia and what to expect as a caregiver. I needed it spelled out that she was dying, and that it was because I loved her that the pain of losing her was so great. The second was a chance to name and explore my grief. I needed a witness to my dark feelings; an understanding and acceptance of the complexity of this relationship and the conflicting feelings. Maybe if those two things had been present, I could have been easier on myself. I loved my mother, and I served her as well as I was able to at the time. I was far from perfect, so far. But I was at her side for the last 10 days of her life. I told her in all honesty what I knew was happening, and my presence gave my sisters the confidence to show up to be with her. We put aside all differences and came together as one as we told her that she was loved. I held her hand and wept as she took her last breath. I wanted to be there, and I felt both genuine compassion and love for her. A kind care aid helped me wash her one last time and anoint her body with oil, my sisters bearing witness, connecting us to all the women throughout time who have attended to their loved ones' bodies.

Sometimes I can picture her exactly as she was before my brother died, before my aunt died, before my dad died, and before dementia. In this picture, she comforts me, she tells me that everything is okay, that she understands. In this picture, she laughs, and I am reminded that for most of my life ... there was love.

CHAPTER EIGHT:
Ongoing professional development is required but not always helpful

Blindsided

Over the years I have attended many, many conferences. I have always been an enthusiastic and prolific presenter, despite experiencing extreme performance anxiety. We are expected, as counsellors, to share our knowledge with other professions, but the combination of presenting and attending workshops can be both tiring and overwhelming. One conference in particular stands out, perhaps because I arrived in a professional mode, but unexpectedly was struck in a very personal way. Here is how it went.

The Volunteer

The conference was called the "Assembly of Grief." It was organized by a number of groups that support the bereaved, and most prominently, by an organization that supports parents whose children have died. I go to several palliative care conferences a year, and I know the pattern of these events. There is a form and a rhythm that I have come to expect: an opening ceremony and address, followed by workshops, breakout groups, and opportunities to network. Conferences, although inspiring, can also be overwhelming, and to counteract the seriousness of our time together, Saturday night often culminates in a gala with some form of entertainment, followed by a live band and dance. I have seen stand-up comics, laugh therapists, bluegrass bands, and a wonderful opera singer and comedian who performed simultaneously in French and English. This type of entertainment provides a much-needed break for both presenters and participants of palliative care conferences. The scheduled singer for Saturday night is a big draw: his music was an influential and delightful soundtrack for my teenage years. I am definitely looking forward to the concert.

My two counselling colleagues, Maria and Allyson, are with me for the opening address. We are seated in a huge auditorium. The lights are dimmed, and only a soft murmur can be heard as we wait expectantly for *something to happen*. Like being seated in a peaceful landscape watching from a distance as a mountain rumbles, there is both excitement and apprehension, when suddenly, music erupts from huge speakers that have been placed around the room, accompanied by colourful, flashing lights that spin around. Startled and a bit alarmed, I do a 360-degree scan and see that towards the back of the hall, there are two people clutching huge bouquets of helium balloons, their arms stretched out in front of them. Back to back, taking short halting steps, they begin to circle the room, with the intention, I gather, to meet again at the front of the hall. I begin to laugh, and turn to my colleagues, but the flashing lights and booming music are so disconcerting that they seem momentarily stunned. The whole scene seems incredibly corny to me.

The song is a lament that asks, "Where have all the balloons gone?" Yet, to my surprise, I notice that, apart from my colleagues and me, everyone is weeping. After the two balloon holders—who I have now dubbed "the robotic brides"—reach the stage, a woman in her late thirties relieves them of their props and gives each a huge hug. All three are weeping. She hands the unruly platoon of balloons to a second person on the stage and, grasping the microphone in both hands, welcomes us by enthusiastically shouting into it, like a cheerleader trying to whip up a crowd. The music fades, and she tearfully and dramatically tells the story of her mother's death when she was a child.

This is a long way from an academic address by a keynote speaker, which I am used to hearing. The dissonance of the balloons and music, reinforced by what feels more like an infomercial than a tragic story, is bewildering. It seems that I am supposed to feel moved, but if anything, I feel the opposite—numb. No, more like ... cold.

As the week progresses, I find out that, unlike the conferences I go to, most people attending are not professionals—not spiritual care providers, counsellors, psychologists, social workers, nurses, doctors, pharmacists, or hospice volunteers—the people who usually attend these events. Other than funeral directors, I don't think I meet any other professionals at all, and only later, when I really need support, do I find a hospice volunteer. The participants are mainly parents of children who have died. The organizers, who are also bereaved parents, apparently were not met in their grief the way that they would have liked, so they thought it would be good to bring professionals together with grieving parents so that the professionals could learn a thing or two. I have a few problems with this.

First, I feel defensive. I'm sorry that they weren't met well, but they are preaching to the choir. I'm sure that I could learn from them, and yet it doesn't seem that they were upfront with this agenda.

The other issue is that I am also a bereaved parent. I really did not expect there to be this kind of focus. I'm in my professional mode, but it's not just that I am unable to switch gears. It's more that I don't want to. Not because I am unwilling to feel or express the grief that I carry, but rather, that this is a venue that does not feel conducive to healing. I feel a bit like I've been duped; called to the principal's office to get a treat, but instead given a lecture, or worse, the strap. However, I must take some responsibility. Most likely, all of this was outlined in the promotional material, and it is possible that I didn't see it, but rather signed up through our education department without thoroughly understanding what was being offered.

The conference continues, and I attend a workshop in which the presenter is against abortion and is talking about the disenfranchised grief of those who have had abortions. Fair enough. But there is an evangelistic quality to her speech that I'm guessing might be well received in certain parts of the United States (where she comes from), but at this conference, which is in Canada, her stance is not at all popular. The workshop participants are uncomfortably silent at first, and then chaos erupts as workshop participants challenge her by asking how she would handle it if her daughter was pregnant and decided to abort. The presenter seems taken aback and can't seem to get back on her feet. I have never heard an anti-abortionist speak in person before, and I am shocked at what I am hearing, and very disturbed by the interchange. Although I have difficulty with the rigidity and lack of compassion in her stance on the issue of abortion, I have tremendous compassion for her as a speaker. I am watching my own worst "presenter nightmare" unfold.

At break times, we are instructed to sit in the large dining hall. Each table has room for about 10 people. Several times a day we introduce ourselves, telling the group what has brought us here. At the first table, before the introductions are in full swing, I am still somewhat naively thinking that I am going to meet others who serve the dying and bereaved. But no, each person has had some horrible tragedy involving their child. One man's son, whom he proudly described as a "superstar," was celebrating his graduation from medical school by going on a hayride with his cohort. Tragically, the wheel fell off, throwing the son to the ground, where a broken spoke punctured his chest and impaled his heart, killing him instantly. Another woman tells of her daughter, who drowned while river rafting in South America.

My daughter has just left for Ecuador for a year of study. After my infant son Dante died, I had resolved not to dwell on my fears of losing another child, but my determination is being challenged as we continue around the table.

One young man killed in a motorcycle accident, a young woman murdered on her first day in Paris, another smashed to pieces when he fell through the roof of a three-storey greenhouse. On and on it goes, story after story. Every meal, every coffee break becomes an ordeal. When I check in with my colleagues, they are struggling, as well. Maria says she is done and leaves the conference.

The schedule is brutal. Speakers are scheduled for first thing in the morning, followed by workshops that begin at 8:30 or 9:00 a.m. and continue all day and late into the evening, with very short breaks for meals or refreshments. To top it off, support groups are scheduled at 10:00 at night, in order to debrief the day and talk about individual losses. When Meadowview is paying for me to be at a conference, I feel an obligation to attend the full session ... but this is too much.

When Saturday night arrives, I am relieved to go to the main hall to hear the music. It begins at 8:00 p.m. Imagine my surprise when the singer gets up, sings three bars of his most popular song, stops abruptly, and says, "Okay now that we have that out of the way, let me tell you about my daughter's suicide." He then goes on to tell the events leading up to his daughter's death, his own retreat into substance abuse, followed by his treatment and recovery. He is still talking at 10:00 p.m. Although it seems incredibly rude, I leave the conference hall.

The next morning, I am looking at the schedule. There is one workshop that has really intrigued me. It is a man who has been contracted by the hospital association in a large city. He is a photographer, and he takes pictures of children who die before or shortly after they are born. It could be because they are premature, stillborn, suffer injury while being born, or during post-natal surgery. Although it seems macabre, it resonates with something in me. When Dante died, I was dismayed to find that we had few pictures of him. It rang true that there might be value in photographing a baby so that the family would have a record that their child had been a part of a family, had been loved. This workshop is scheduled for the afternoon.

Meanwhile, I find a truly wonderful offering; a moment of relief in the fast lane to despair. It is given by a music therapist who has brought a huge collection of singing bowls gathered from around the world. Singing bowls produce sounds that summon a deep state of relaxation, naturally assisting the listener to enter a meditative state, and they are believed to aid in relaxation, healing, and perhaps enlightenment. Many people find that the rich blend of harmonic overtones that the bells produce have a direct affect upon their ability to clear and centre their energy.

The therapist asks if someone would be willing to come to the front so that she can demonstrate. Several people wave their hands, and she selects a man who agrees to lie on the carpeted floor while the other participants gather in a circle around him. The presenter outlines his shape by placing the bowls a few inches from his body, so that he is completely surrounded by them. She then sets the bowls ringing, explaining that she can hear, by the tone of the sound, when a person's energy is blocked. By continuing to play a bowl where there is resistance, she can move the person's energy. The man obviously experiences the treatment as extremely relaxing, although he uses the word "blissful." For those of us watching, it is a sacred moment of healing, as we allow the ancient sounds of the bowls to penetrate our beings. What a gift!

In the break, rather than sit at another table with more parents, I go out onto the lawn and stretch out, my face pressed into the grass. I am overcome with emotion and collapse into big sobs. I feel incredibly lonely. I wish that I had a friend to talk to, and I long for my husband. I want to melt into his arms and cry. I want to hold my kids tightly and burrow my face into them, inhale their scent. I want to be reassured that death is not around every corner, waiting to grab them.

After a while, my thoughts drift and I am thinking about what would happen if my husband were to die. From there, I think about travelling. Could I go off on my own, like I did when I was 18? I can remember being young and feeling the same kind of desperate loneliness that I am feeling now. It seems that so much of our sense of identity is rooted in being known; in shared understanding of the world, and where we fit into that world. Who am I if no one recognizes me? But does it have to be like that, I wonder?

A vivid picture occurs to me. I am back in the London of my youth, and in my fantasy, I approach someone on the street, or maybe on a bench, and I strike up a conversation. I say, "I'm feeling really lonely and homesick." Would he or she be empathetic? If someone came up to me and said that, I think that I would try to comfort them. In fact, I remember a time when I saw a woman at an airport crying into her hands. I went over to her and put my arm around her. She continued crying, and when she stopped, she thanked me profusely. I never even found out what was upsetting her. I was a stranger, and I responded. I come out of my reverie and think, "Okay, I am that woman, and I need help."

First, I go looking for my colleague Allyson, but I cannot find her. I sit on one of the couches in the lobby, trying to decide what to do, when a man comes and sits beside me. He introduces himself as a volunteer from a hospice on one of the nearby islands. He appears to be so solid and present that, without much hesitation, I just jump in and say, "I'm having a really hard time." I let out a huge breath and start to cry. "It's just that I feel so overwhelmed right now ... and really, really lonely." There. I have said it. He responds warmly, with interest. Before long, I feel much better. We talk for a while, and then he asks me which workshop I am going to. I tell him that I had wanted to hear the man who photographs families after their child dies, but I am feeling so raw that I'm not sure if I can go. I tell him about Dante's death, and how this particular presentation might be very difficult for me.

"I would be happy to go with you, if that would help," he kindly offers.

"Okay ..." I hesitate, feeling anxious, but at the same time relieved that I don't have to miss it.

We move to the front of a small, darkened classroom with about 20 others. The presenter's photography work had begun when he was invited to go to the local hospital by a concerned nurse who had experienced two late miscarriages. Her own experience had led her to institute a bereavement program in the neonatal unit where she worked. She had invited him to take photographs as part of a plan to help the neonatal program staff be more responsive to the needs of bereaved parents. Moving away from the tradition of whisking a baby away without letting the mother see it, in this program, mothers could hold their babies, family were welcome, and nurses took photographs. The families were appreciative of this loving attitude, and she could see how much more healing it was for them. She then got permission to invite a professional photographer to take the photos.

His first response was dismay. Photographing dead babies? Then he began researching the subject, and found out that there was a long history of photographing the dead, evidenced by the beautiful daguerreotypes from the 1800s that he found at flea markets. He began his slide show with a selection of daguerreotypes showing families seated in formal poses. In every slide, there was a dead child among the other family members. In some photos the child is laid out, but more often, he or she is seated among the family, dressed in fine clothing.

After a similar slide show of paintings through the ages, the presenter tentatively, sensitively, and with great respect eases us towards his work. He explains that, when the staff at this particular hospital sees that a baby is likely to die or has just died, the family is asked if they would like a photographer to attend. Surprisingly, many families agree. He brings his equipment, and after making a connection with family members, he melds into the background, shooting photos. He then creates an album of about 50 8-by-10 photographs that document the child with his or her family. After about a month, he contacts the family and spends an evening or an afternoon going through the album with them.

The photos are exquisite. Somehow, he is able to transcend a horrendous scene—a stark stainless-steel operating room, twisted blankets half off the table, equipment strewn on the counters—and finds the mother holding the tiniest wrapped bundle, with a perfect hand or foot exposed, the family leaning in, tremendous love and sorrow evident on their faces. He captures intimate moments of exquisite tenderness: the softest brush of lips on the downy back of a premature child ... a stillborn baby perfect in every way, dressed in a lacy christening gown.

The emotional impact of seeing these photos is beautifully balanced with the phenomenal compassion and sensitivity of the photographer and the obvious value of his work. I am deeply moved, silently crying. It is not a bad feeling, like the despair that I had felt earlier, but softer, a feeling of unity rather than isolation; a sense of connection to all humans who grieve. By the time he explains that, for some families his photographs are the only record of the child, I think everyone in the room is sold on the idea.

As I sit in the darkened room, watching the slides, listening to the speaker and crying, I glance over at the volunteer who has accompanied me to the presentation, and I notice that in the empty seat between us, he has placed his upturned hand. It is an offer of support, should I want it. Silently, I slide over beside him and take his hand. I feel comforted. When the speaker is finished and we stand up to clap, the volunteer puts his arms around me and holds me tightly to his chest as I sob.

I learned some important lessons that week. Preconceptions colour how we experience an event. I was unable to shake the feeling that the organizers had an agenda. My back was up, and my heels dug in. Had I known that agenda, I would not have attended. Had the workshops been designed for dialogue, where there was a chance for professionals to be heard and supported as well as educated, then I may have received their message more readily.

The second lesson had to do with the scheduling of the workshops. It was overwhelming, and not conducive to healing or growth. It was not stressed enough that we were meant to choose, or to be selective, but rather, there seemed to be an expectation that we would attend the entire program. Of course, it was up to each of us to care for ourselves, but I think that, as professionals, when organizing an event, we must be realistic about what people can take in at any given time—especially vulnerable people.

Early in my career as a child protection social worker, I had attended a conference on sexual abuse. One day at lunchtime, the scheduled speaker was going to talk about a very heavy topic: ritual abuse. If you are lucky enough not to know what that is, suffice it to say that it was an alleged form of physical and sexual abuse, mainly of children, by satanic cults. It was subsequently discredited, but at the time, it seemed very real.

I like to think that the organizers simply made a mistake in the timing. The speaker began as the wait staff were serving dessert, a creamy yellow pudding with a blob of strawberry jam in the middle, which looked a lot like a splotch of blood. As the speaker told horrendous stories of torture and torment of young children, the young waiters and waitresses continued to collect glasses and whisper into participants' ears, "Coffee, tea?" Were we really expected to eat pudding while listening to the speaker? I felt concerned for the young servers, wondering what it was like for them to hear these horrendous tales. Even for me, a seasoned social worker, it was highly disturbing. I would have to have been completely dissociated to eat the rest of my lunch. Ironically, that was the point the speaker was making: that children survived overwhelming situations by separating from their bodies, turning to substance abuse, and later in life, not being able to recognize or extract themselves from unhealthy situations.

I vowed then that I would never speak under circumstances that were so dissonant to healing. When designing workshops, we must take into consideration the space and timing of emotionally charged subjects, and we must model self-care, which means providing a safe environment in which participants are able to process what they are seeing, thinking, feeling and hearing.

I also began to get a glimpse of what self-care really means. I think that I can justifiably say that the workshop was not well organized, and that the situation itself was stressful. I can say that I didn't get enough rest. I can say that I did not attend to my emotions. My time at the conference was not balanced among physical, emotional, spiritual, social and mental activities. The palliative care literature defines palliative care as a stressful occupation, and tries to support us by providing suggestions on how to reduce stress: physical activity, fresh air, solid sleep, a healthy diet, time with friends, listening to music, and prayer or meditation. Had I done any of these things, I would have felt better, I'm sure. However, I probably would not have spent much time at the conference.

For some people, the conference may not have been stressful at all. By framing it as "stressful," or "not well organized," I place the blame and the responsibility of my stress on the situation or the organization. That perspective doesn't help me in the moment, and most likely won't help me or anyone else in the long term. For example, to feel better, I would have had to convince the organizers that they were in the wrong to have organized the conference in the way that they did. If they hadn't agreed, I would have felt frustrated and angry, and possibly bitter, if I had put a lot of energy into my argument.

To frame my stress as due to a "lack of balance" blames me for my own stress and suggests that I need to be fixed or improved in some way. I think that there is a better way to understand this. While the suggestions offered by the literature on how to combat stress and burnout provide good strategies, they are just not effective when we apply them randomly. To be effective in any situation, self-care needs to be in response to an experience, not just applied willy-nilly. Tuning into one's own body, noticing emotions and identifying needs is more likely to be effective. We cannot expect other people—whether friends, family, co-workers or managers—to know what we are feeling and needing. Once we articulate for ourselves what we are feeling, then we are more likely to know what we need.

It seems that things got better for me when I attended the music workshop and calmed myself. Then, by taking some time alone to let myself feel the uncomfortable and perhaps unwelcome feelings of loneliness and despair, I was able to identify what I needed, and to find someone with whom I could connect. I realize now that self-care is about taking our own experience seriously, without criticism, and then responding appropriately. If we ignore or dismiss our bodily sensations or our feelings, or if we respond to needs such as sleep, hunger, danger or loneliness with dissonant strategies, such as alcohol, food or more activity, we are guilty of disrespect, and we cause our own suffering. First, we need to be attuned and honest with ourselves.

Many people really like to help. But I think that the true test of one's character is whether, we—especially caregivers—can accept help. Yes, I felt vulnerable asking for help. Maybe the volunteer wondered if he would be adequate for my request, and when he reached out his hand, he felt vulnerable too. Neither of us knew what would happen. Yet somehow, we both took a chance. We both must have believed, even for a moment, that connection is possible, even with a stranger.

And that is the other lesson: there *are* good people, sometimes found randomly, who will notice that another person is in distress, and who will take a chance and reach out a hand. All we have to do is accept it.

CHAPTER NINE:
When professional development really helps

The Essential Space Between Theory and Reality

For caregivers, providing palliative care is creative balance between what we can know—from theory, developing our skills, and experience—and what we will never know: how this particular patient or family member will respond in this particular setting, at this particular time, to these particular people and to death. To imagine differently is a dangerous practice, because it gives us false confidence, implying that we can anticipate and know what we or another person will feel or do.

For example, in health care, our models, protocols and best practices imply that we can imagine and have imagined the possibilities of what might occur, and that the model or protocol is providing not only appropriate responses, but the best responses which will then become standard. The individual caregiver or team can follow these steps and be confident that they are doing or getting it right. But we know that, in facing death, real life does not work like that. We can know what some of the hazards of encountering mortality might be through our theoretical knowledge of providing palliative care, and we can know how we have responded to mortality in the past, but we can never know what a particular encounter with mortality will stir in us. We cannot prevent our own suffering by prescribing either a prophylactic that diverts or transforms unpleasant feelings, or a salve to treat feelings after the fact, any more than we can prevent suffering in our patients. There are far too many shifting variables within our own beings, and in the world in which we interact, for us to be able to accurately anticipate our own thoughts, feelings and actions.

Counselling is more an art than a skill, although skills are certainly involved. But because of the complexity of human beings, and the myriad ways to encounter death, there is no real way to learn the art without just jumping in and doing the work. While being educated in counselling skills and embracing palliative care philosophy can form the basis for helping others, there can be no scripts. In *Finite and Infinite Games*, religious scholar James Carse (1986) writes that, in the game of life, learning requires the players to be prepared to be surprised by the future, which requires complete openness. He is referring here not to candour, but to allowing ourselves to be vulnerable, to be open to metamorphosis. Because of the complexity of human nature, then, contrary to the medical model, when it comes to dealing with people and their emotions, there can never be pre-planned scripts or "best practices."

In other words, there is no way to anticipate what others will say or do, but even more importantly, there is no way to anticipate what we ourselves will say and do in any given situation. Even so, complexity theory tells us that there is more to understand than the complexity of each individual's unique and changing living system. Each person is attached to other individual living systems that are similarly changing, and those individuals are embedded in other changing systems. Without taking into consideration the complexity and the spontaneous, evolving elements of any situation, any plan that we make provides false assurance that we will know what to do in a given situation.

Our theories and models of palliative care, together with our values, are the foundation of hospice work, but there will always be a space between what we can know theoretically and the moment-to-moment experience of encountering mortality. From my perspective, the gap between what we can know and what there is to know is not a flaw in our knowledge, but rather an essential part of the complex nature of what it means to be human.

In the following story, I find myself in a situation that clearly could never have been anticipated.

The Family Conference

The home care nurse calls to tell us that she is at the home of a woman named Janet, and she is finding the situation more than she can handle. She wonders if we can visit, despite it being only an hour before my nursing partner Lee's shift change. The home care nurse describes a complicated family system with years of discord; one sister suffering from depression after her husband's death, another with a mentally challenged child, and a brother who has only recently reconciled with the family.

Lee and I head over to Janet's house. The day has been extremely hectic, with call after call, but Lee and I have managed. We work really well together. For me, it can be a joy to work so closely with my nursing partner, and because Lee and I work together regularly, we have established a solid rhythm. Working with people from different disciplines, which is a reality for our team, creates both rewards and challenges. We have to learn to work with different agendas, styles and responsibilities. Lee and I have learned how to move seamlessly from being the leader to the follower, as the situation requires. We are used to sensing our way through situations, attuned to slight nuances in each other's speech and demeanour. It's like dancing: sometimes the beat is slow and the steps easy to follow, while at other times, the music takes us on crazy bends and turns, spinning us around, so that following the steps becomes almost impossible, and the dance becomes pure intuition. At other times, we seemingly dance solo, but we each know that we are most definitely not alone, and in those times, we need to be even more in sync with each other. I really like the feeling of connection and attunement that we share, as once again we enter the unknown.

We step up to the small front porch, trying to balance all of our bags and supplies. Lee uses her elbow to lift the door knocker, and it falls with a thud. A tired-looking, dishevelled woman cracks the door open and peeks through. After we introduce ourselves, she opens the door and tells us that her name is Julia, Janet's sister. She ushers us in, trying to keep a fluffy black cat and a small, yapping dog from escaping. I am fairly sensitive to smells at the best of times, but nothing has prepared me for the wall of hot, rank odour that I must step through. The smell of urine and feces is overwhelming. I seriously consider turning around and walking back to the car. Irrationally, I take a deep breath and hold it as I follow Julia to Janet's bedroom.

Julia and her younger sister Janice hover over Janet, and we watch for a minute before joining them at the bedside. Julia is trembling as she tearfully gives us some background. Lee then offers to examine Janet, and I step into the hall with Julia. Julia is distraught because she thinks that she has made a mistake in not insisting that Janet be provided with a feeding tube. Now that the end is nearing, she desperately wants to buy more time. I acknowledge how frightening it must be to see her sister like this and explore the feeling that she should be doing something. I explain that when a person is dying, their whole system begins to slow, and they are unable to digest food, eliminate waste, or to even process water. We find that if fluids are given, they go into the tissues, creating swelling, and most often, into the lungs, which ends up as pneumonia. The good part is that nature has arranged it so that most dying people do not experience any hunger or thirst.

Julia seems reassured that she has indeed made the right decision.

She then asks me if I will see her brother, who seems to be struggling. She sends Janice to the basement to see if John will speak to me. He comes upstairs immediately, and I am taken to the large dining room table. Once again, the smell is overpowering, and I feel like I am being smothered. That, added to the oppressing tension that blankets the house, is nauseating. As I pull out a chair to sit down, I am shocked to see the source of the horrible stench. Someone has built a shallow plywood box that sits on the floor at the base of the table. It is the entire size of the table, and it is filled with fine gravel that serves as a huge litter box for the numerous animals in the house. Neither John nor his sisters give any indication that they notice the smell or the disgusting visual. In self-defence, I place my hand over my mouth and nose in what I am hoping is a casual posture, as I take a seat and attempt to focus my attention on John.

He is eager to talk. His dad died when he was six years old, and his mom married a man who, according to John, "has not been a good father." John elaborates in some detail about being beaten repeatedly throughout his childhood, despite his continued efforts to earn his stepfather's love. One day, John tells me, he just couldn't take it anymore: he hit back and left the house. He had no contact with the family for many years. Tearfully, he relates that on the day he left, he lost "everything," and thought that he would never see his family again. But then a few years ago, his mother had contacted him and asked for his help. John nursed her until her death and has continued to live in the basement. His stepdad now has dementia, and although John tells him daily that he has a job and has had continuous work for the past 20 years, his stepdad still believes that John is unemployed and will never amount to much. Now John's main priority is for his sister to be allowed to die in peace. He also wants his stepfather to be placed in long-term care, and the family pet, a dying pig named Dawg, taken to the vet and put to sleep. There seem to be multiple issues for everyone in the family.

I ask all of the siblings to join me in the living room for a meeting. As I enter, the first thing I notice is Dawg the pig, a small, hairless bundle that is trembling so badly that she can hardly stand, looking at me with wild, frightened eyes. I have no idea how to respond, but once again, I feel sick. Beyond the dying pig, I see the stepfather in his big recliner. When I introduce myself, he stares back blankly. Janice coaches him to stand up, accompanying him as he unsteadily shuffles into a back bedroom. Janice comes back and scoops up Dawg, disappearing again. When she returns, the other family members and Lee take their places on the chairs that have been set up in a circle.

I feel unsure of how to proceed. How will I cut through the heavy tension that sits upon us all? It is hard to sort out the volume of issues before me, so I focus on my own feelings, trying to calm and settle myself. I begin by saying that there are some things that need to be discussed. My intention is to draw on my recent training with educator and author Marshall Rosenberg's work in nonviolent communication. But first, I decide to talk about talking about it.

"Before we get to the hard stuff," I say, "I would like for each of you to take a turn to tell me what you think is the most important thing about how we conduct this meeting." I am met by silence. So, after a moment has passed, I turn to Janice. "Janice, what is the most important thing to you?"

As I go around the room, there is intense emotion and an urgency to tell stories of communication that has been unclear, painful and incomplete. Perhaps somewhat awkwardly, I attempt, as per Rosenberg, to translate each statement that includes blame and labelling, into unmet needs. I ask each person if there is anything more that they want to say, but miraculously, each one says that they feel that they have been heard. I then thank them for being so honest and clear about what they need. I summarize, reinforcing that they actually are in complete agreement that they would all like to be heard, they want clear and complete information, they want respect, and they want to come to agreement about some important decisions that have to be made.

I then ask them what they would like to talk about. John jumps in, saying that he is "sick and tired of Julia being some sort of Mother Teresa—she's not the only person who cares about Janet." I continue to translate his feelings into needs.

"So, you're feeling frustrated because you'd like some recognition that you care about Janet too."

"Yes." That is it. And he doesn't want some big, phony funeral. Again, I respond by acknowledging that he is feeling worried, because he wants there to be open communication and shared decision making.

"Yes." That is it. I ask him what he would like to see happen.

Well, he wants her to be cremated, because that is what she said that she wanted, and that's what she had decided for their mom when she died. John wants her ashes thrown to the wind.

"It's important to you that things are kept simple, and that your sister's wishes are honoured," I reiterate.

"Yes." That's what he needs.

I move to Julia. "Julia, can you tell me what you would like to talk about?"

She is furious ... furious because she is sick and tired of her brother yelling at her. He is always yelling. He can't say anything without yelling. She loves her family, and it is so painful to her that they are all screaming at each other. She knows that her sister would feel so pained to know that they are out here fighting while she is dying.

Taking a deep breath, I translate her concerns into needs. "It's really important to you that there is respect and a sense of being together ... of harmony."

"Yes." I am correct.

Since she is the executrix, she has decided that her sister will be cremated, and a stone will be placed in the cemetery, which is what Julia had done when her husband died.

"For you, then, it's important to have a place that you can return to," I say, in an effort to subtly move away from solutions and strategies. I am trying to make it clear that this is Julia's opinion, and not a done deal. I continue around the room until I am able to summarize that they agree about the cremation, followed by a simple service.

It is brought forward that they have not settled on where the ashes will be spread. I take them through another round and establish that they agree about having a place to return to. They quickly identify a lake that they had visited with their grandparents, agreeing that they will scatter Janet's ashes in this lake after the service.

Janice's issue has to do with whether or not to give Janet some medication that will dry up the secretions in her throat. This is a highly charged issue, as Janet has heart problems that developed after she took a cold remedy. Janice is concerned that the proposed medicine will speed up Janet's heart and hasten her death. John and Julia think that the congestion should be managed. More animated discussion ensues, about whether she should be turned on her side or on her back. Lee goes over the pros and cons of both the medication and the turning. At some point, they reach an agreement to hold the medication, but to turn her regularly. By the end of the conversation, however, they collectively change their minds and decide to allow Lee to administer the drug.

We go through the same process to decide who will arrange for the pig to be taken to the vet, who will contact the funeral home, who will write the obituary, and who will arrange for the eulogy. Two hours have passed, and everyone, including me, is exhausted, so I suggest that we close the meeting. To my utter amazement, Julia asks if we can have a group hug, to which everyone agrees. They express appreciation for our team, and we leave.

As it turns out, Lee and I are on the next day. Lee, who starts her shift before I do, receives a frantic phone call from Julia. She says that John is getting angry and threatening to karate-kick her. Lee advises her to call the police. Julia apparently does this, telling the dispatcher that her brother is being violent and is out of control, to which the dispatcher responds by sending a police officer. That is, until the second call, shortly afterward, when Julia frantically and somewhat abruptly reports that her sister is dead. The dispatcher assumes that the two calls are related and dispatches the SWAT team, in addition to the police officer. Julia also phones Lee back, and Lee calls me to ask if she can pick me up from my house so that we get to Janet's house more quickly.

We arrive to see an ambulance, a police wagon and several police cars with doors open and lights flashing. John is face down on the grass, his hands cuffed behind his back, surrounded by police officers in full combat gear. Lee proceeds immediately into the house. I linger on the front lawn and get the story from one of the officers. John is subdued, but crying. He does not seem to be a threat at this point, so I kneel down beside him and put my arms around him. I stroke his hair as he sobs and chokes out his story. He expresses his fury at his sister. "She was so obviously dying, and she just wouldn't take care of it." He is crying so hard that he can no longer speak, but after a while, he sobs, "I just didn't want her to suffer."

I'm a little confused. Is he talking about the pig or his sister? The police officer witnesses our exchange and unlocks the handcuffs. Lee addresses the officer's questions inside the house, explaining that this is an expected death, so there is no need to call the coroner. That's the last thing we need. The police leave, and I suggest that we all move into the living room.

I am reminded of my own family at the time my mother was diagnosed with dementia. Early on, before she completely lost touch with reality and before her long slide towards death, much like this family, my siblings and I were struggling to agree on even the simplest things. One morning I awoke, shaken, from a dream in which I was happily walking in the countryside. The sun was shining. I could see a sparkling ocean in the distance. There were wildflowers everywhere. I was startled when something flew by my face, brushing my cheek. I kept walking, but before long, I realized that there were small missiles coming at me from all directions. Suddenly, I was struck. I saw that it was a needle that had entered my arm and disappeared. I looked up to see that there were snipers peeking out everywhere, with weapons akin to machine guns, but loaded with needles. I realized, with horror, that the needle had entered my bloodstream and was travelling towards my heart. I knew that I would be wounded for the rest of my life. "What could it mean?" I remember laughing to a friend when I told her the dream.

It seems like I have returned to the family battle-field. John is glaring at Julia, and every time she looks up, he lets out a low, throaty growl, raises his fist and, leaning towards her, half-sitting, half-standing, he gives her the finger. 'Okay', I think to myself, 'I need to be more directive here'. Despite my success last night, I am doubtful of my ability to go forward. I look to Lee, and she gives me a reassuring look. This is a situation in which I may *appear* to be dancing alone. While I am clearly in charge of the family meeting, I am extremely conscious of Lee's silent support. I know that she is with me and will step in to catch me if I stumble.

Once again, I identify feelings and try to trans-late what each person is saying into unmet needs. I acknowledge that there are intense feelings right now and make a point of not singling out any one person. I address everyone in the group, telling them that I would really appreciate it if they would please hang in with me so that we can make the decisions that have to be made.

I draw on my crisis training, which is to focus only on what needs to be decided *now*. Amazingly, I am able to get each person to agree to a plan for themselves. Julia will go to an appointment that was previously set with her counsellor. Janice will call the funeral home and make appropriate arrangements. John is going to take some space and try to calm himself. I refer them to family counseling and victim services, as the police recommended, and I wind up our visit. Lee and I return to the unit, where we meet with other staff to debrief before carrying on with the rest of our day.

I continue to think of Julia, Janice and John. Despite their difficulties, love was there. They showed up, they were trying. I wonder if the experience of a family meeting in which they were each heard had any impact. I hope that they have put down their rifles and stopped sniping at each other. I hope they have stopped the needling. I want, for their sakes, for the war to end, for them to learn to communicate in a way that helps them connect, and for them to find the love for which they yearn. Each one of them is responsible for creating this toxic situation. It is so easy to blame other people; to be so sure that the other person is the one causing problems. The real work begins when we start to think about our own contribution, and the impact of our own words and actions. I only know this because I lived it myself. It has taken me a long time to lay down my own weapons. The poet Rumi (1997) says, "Your task is not to seek for love, but merely to seek and find all the barriers within yourself that you have built against it" (np).

CHAPTER TEN:
This is why we stay

At the Heart of Palliative Care

In their article, "Words" in the *Journal of Research in Personality*, University of Texas professors Carla Groom and James Pennebaker (2002) observed that, "Words are the building blocks of meaning, social interaction, and language itself. The ways people speak say a lot about who they are" (p.615-621). Where I worked in palliative care, when a person dies or is about to die, we used the words "dying," "die," "death" or "dead." For example, we might say to a patient's family member, "Your father will most likely die in the next few hours," or "Your mother is dead"; or to the patient, "What would you like to happen to your body after you die?" This direct speech must be understood in the context of the larger hospice/palliative care movement, which avoids euphemistic terms that replace a word such as "died," which can seem stark or harsh, with a less offensive (but also less accurate or descriptive) term, such as "passed away," "gone," or "gone to Heaven." By being specific in saying, "We think that your mother is actively dying and has hours to days to live," we can be much clearer than if we say, for example, "Your mother is nearing the end of her life," or "Your mother's time is short." Although these words can be hard for a family member to hear, for some it is helpful to know that "a short time" is not a few years, or even a few months. Practising direct speech reflects and reinforces our mandate and our intention to provide clear, accurate and complete information to patients and their families, and is understood to be an invitation and a model for others to speak openly with us.

Contrary to popular opinion, this approach is even more important when it comes to children. By being direct and forthcoming, children learn to trust their parents and trust that they will keep them informed and will tell the truth. By opening up the subject, they are able to understand why emotions are escalated, and they are then able to go through a grieving process in step with the adults around them, rather than after the fact.

Information goes a long way in preparing everybody. In this final story, we see the value of providing clear information, in the sense that both the patient and her family can now make decisions knowing that these are the "last times"—that she will leave the house, that she will go outside, that they will have the privacy to say what is in their hearts.

I think that this story also captures the quint-essential values of palliative care: to make a connection, to allow space, to provide information as needed, to show compassion, and to be guided by the patient and family. It's the impression that I most want to savour. Here it is.

When Time Stops

"Ah," I sigh, as Joanne and I settle into the car, "don't you just love the feeling of driving away?"

"Yeah," she says, rolling down the window.

"We're so free ... if the nurses on the unit only knew how great our job is, they'd all want to work on our team. I'm so glad I'm not stuck inside all the time," I say, smiling as I move the car through the parking area and into light morning traffic. It's a beautiful day. The rhododendrons that surround the parking lot at Meadowview Hospice are in full bloom. It strikes me that the way the sun is shining behind them makes the deep cadmium red look as if it is reaching out towards us, demanding that we take notice. 'I see you', I say to myself, and almost laugh out loud.

After making our way through the commercial area of town, we head for the suburbs. Breaking the comfortable silence between us, I ask Joanne what she knows about our next visit. Too late, I notice that she has her eyes closed and her head back, obviously enjoying the cool air that is ruffling the wispy curls around her face.

"Oh, right," she murmurs. Shoot, I probably should have stayed quiet and let her rest. Not only do nurses work 12-hour shifts, half of their shifts are days and the other half are nights, which wreaks havoc with their circadian rhythms. *And* they are expected to start their shift early to *hear* others report, and stay late, to *give* their reports, as if 12 hours isn't a long enough shift. I usually try to do small things to make their time go a bit easier. But I've interrupted her now; nothing I can do about it.

I have read the pink sheets, which are the psychosocial notes that are primarily written by counsellors describing the social, emotional and spiritual concerns of patients and families, and the reports of previous visits, but I've forgotten what I read. Joanne opens the chart that has been lying on her lap and gives me the quick version.

Helen is an 80-year-old woman who lives part of the year in Toronto, and the rest of the time here, with her son and his family. She arrived about 10 days ago and seemed to be perfectly well: out driving with her grandchildren, meeting a friend at a restaurant, helping her daughter-in-law in the garden. Then, a few nights ago, she went to bed early, saying that she was tired. In the morning, she was too weak to get out of bed. She was sent to Emergency where, after a series of tests, she was told that she had an aggressive cancer and was within weeks of death. Helen was sent home, because she wanted to take care of some business. The home care nurse who made the referral had told Joanne earlier this morning that Helen had attended to her banking, her will, and her funeral plans and was now asking to be admitted to Meadowview Hospice.

"So," says Joanne, "we need to check her out and see if it's an appropriate referral."

"Can you imagine? Your mom comes to stay, you're expecting to have a wonderful time. Your kids are all hyped up about grandma coming—and then this?" Even though I've been working at hospice for a long time, I am still amazed at how quickly someone's world can change.

"Yeah," she says, "and when she left her home, she didn't know that it would be the last time she would see her house and her friends ..." We both take a minute to imagine that.

"What gets me is that she seems to have just accepted that this is the way it is," I add incredulously.

"That's what the home care nurse said," agrees Joanne, "although she may have had a sense that something was wrong, I suppose."

"Maybe ..."

We fall into silence again. I wonder if I can be as gracious as Helen when my time comes. I envision being at my doctor's office. It's James, my doctor for the past 30 years. He's gentle, maybe even tearful. "Okay, I'm ready," I say bravely.

Nope. That will never happen. I'm just not the kind of person who accepts things. I'd fight.

"How would you handle it, if you were Helen?" I ask Joanne.

"I'd like to say that I would just know, and give in ... but probably not. It would be a wonderful gift though, to your family, to just surrender and show them that there's nothing to be afraid of."

"Yeah." In another Walter Mitty moment, I imagine myself lying at hospice—no, in my own bed—my family around me crying, and I am reassuring them that it's all okay.

"Mm, I think I'm going to have to work on being gracious," I say.

The distance between street signs has grown as we travel the rural route. I see the sign I'm looking for and ask Joanne for the street number. I see it up ahead. Turning into a steep driveway that curves into a forest, the house out of sight from the street, I drive slowly.

"What a gorgeous view," Joanne gushes as we drive through a copse of maples.

When I see the river in the distance, I blurt out, "I'm just so happy." I stop the car on a huge paved area in front of an oversized garage.

"No need to worry about whether there are enough parking spaces," laughs Joanne. I turn the car around so that it is pointing towards the driveway, a habit from being the driver at night. Although it's early in the day, and there's not a huge chance that we will be here until nightfall, we never know. I back up ever so slowly.

"Sorry," I laugh. "If I'm going to go over the edge, I prefer to do it carefully."

As we get out of the car, the mood changes, and we each retreat into ourselves as we walk to the front door. A handsome man, maybe in his fifties, dressed in a loose Hawaiian shirt, answers our knock and introduces himself as David. "And this is my daughter Andrea," he says proudly pointing to the smaller of two petite, red-haired girls who are also dressed in Hawaiian-themed clothes. "She's seven." "This one is Cathy," he says, indicating the taller of the two.

"I'm older," she says.

"Oh, how old are you then?" I ask.

"Ten."

"Nice to meet you Cathy," I say, as I reach out to grasp her small hand. Joanne shakes hands with the others.

David leads the way to the living room, where a hospital bed has been set up. The two girls push past us and take positions at either side of their grand-mother's bed. Andrea has dragged a footstool next to the bed, climbed up and is standing on the far side. She lays her face next to Helen's on the pillow. Cathy stands solemnly to the side. The blankets are immaculately tucked in, Helen's hair is neatly combed, and her hands are folded on her chest.

"You must be Helen," Joanne says warmly. Helen nods.

"I'm nurse Joanne, and this is my partner Susan, she's the counsellor," she says, nodding her chin in my direction. "We are from hospice." She pauses a minute to see how that piece of information lands. Sometimes we walk into homes where they are not expecting us or haven't been told that we are from hospice. Although most people are grateful to see us, some people find our presence frightening at first. This family seems to be prepared for us.

"The home care nurse asked us to come and see how you are doing," Joanne continues.

Helen's arms lift slightly from the bed, as if it is just too much to lift them any higher. Joanne steps closer to grasp each of Helen's hands in her own.

"It sounds like you've had a pretty rough time of it in the last few days."

Helen gives a half-smile and attempts to nod her head.

"You seem tired. Would you like us to talk to your son to get some of the background ... so you can save your energy?" she asks kindly. A look of relief passes briefly across Helen's face, but she says nothing. "Would you like us to have this discussion in the other room, or would you rather we stay in here so that you can hear?"

"In here, please," Helen croaks.

Okay, we know that she is conscious and oriented and can still communicate. She appears pale, but with a slight rosiness high on her cheeks. I can see by the effort it takes to speak that she is extremely weak. David leads us to the couches, where we arrange our bags on the floor and settle in.

"Girls," he says with authority, "please go out onto the patio, and I'll be out in a while."

I am surprised that they leave without a fuss. David fills us in on the past two weeks: how well she seemed when she arrived, how quickly she changed, and the subsequent visit to the hospital. "Mom wants to be at Meadowview at the ..." he pauses, darting a glance in Helen's direction, "... at the end."

"Okay," Joanne and I say in unison.

"She's very close to the girls, but she wants to spare them ... uh ... she's always been quite private." He seems about to say something else, but doesn't finish his sentence, just looks sadly towards Helen. She silently meets his gaze.

"I wonder if it would be alright for me to check you over, take a few vitals, that sort of thing?" Joanne says to Helen.

"How about if David and I go into another room and give you two some privacy," I say to Helen.

"Yes, that would be good," she whispers.

David and I head into the kitchen, where he pulls out a chair for me. I find out that his wife has gone to fill a prescription, but I'm guessing that she may be taking a break in order to compose herself. Jane has been very close to Helen and is struggling to take in the shocking news that Helen is "nearing the end," as David puts it. The family had last seen her in Hawaii where, according to David, Helen had even gone snorkelling with the girls, much to everyone's delight.

"Ah," I say, nodding at his shirt.

"Yup, we all got one," David says wryly. Then turning more serious, he says wistfully, "She adores the girls.".

"It sounds like your mom has been a big part of this family," I say, resting my hand on David's forearm. Reaching for my hand, he takes it, and looks soulfully into my eyes. His eyes fill with tears. There are no words. After a while, I ask him how he feels about Helen going to hospice. He says that he and Jane have talked about it. They both agree that they would happily care for her at home, but it is her wish that she goes to hospice. They want whatever she wants. I talk about there being no right way to go through this, and I describe the unit a bit, since he has never been there.

Our unit is a 10-bed hospice on the hospital grounds. Four of our beds are for people who are living in the community, at home, but who need to come in either because our team has been unable to manage their symptoms at home, or because the home care nurse or physician has established that they need to come to hospice to get their medications sorted out. The plan is that these patients will come for about five to seven days and then return home. We have one respite bed that is for a planned stay of one week, to give either the patient or the family a break, or both. The other five beds are for people in about the last six weeks of their lives. These people come to hospice with no plan of returning home, and they expect to die at hospice.

Despite what many people believe—that hospice is a sad place—most are surprised to find that it is a homey, loving place. There is laughter. There is a sense of safety and often relief when people arrive. Sometimes, people are afraid when they come, but most often they settle in and are glad that they came. Although Meadowview is now dated, it is still better than many hospitals, because most of the rooms are private, there are refrigerators in each room, telephones and music players, and people can bring their own art, pajamas and bedding. Volunteers are available from 7:30 in the morning until 11:00 at night, ready to find a newspaper, make a pot of tea, sit with a lonely person, and answer call bells. There are counsellors available from 9:00 in the morning until around 11:00 at night, as well as a professional spiritual care provider at various times of the day, and many specially trained volunteers who cover the in-patient unit from 7:00 a.m. to 11:00 p.m. At hospice, the family and the patient are cared for.

"The staff at Meadowview is particularly kind and attentive," I tell David. I don't say why I think this is true, but I do believe that we have an advantage over other areas of the medical system, because of the values around emotional support for both staff and the people we serve. That is embedded into our organization.

After a while, I suggest that we see how Joanne is doing with his mom. We walk tentatively back into the living room, not wanting to disturb either a physical examination or an intimate discussion. But Helen is neatly tucked in, and Joanne is seated near her, making notes.

"So, what have you found out?" I ask. Joanne waits until David and I are seated, and then says, "Helen, is it okay with you if I fill them in on our conversation?"

Helen moves her chin slightly, indicating that it is okay.

"Helen is very weak, and she is finding it hard to swallow. She hasn't had any food or water in the last few days, and her chest is beginning to fill with fluid. From what I am seeing, I think that her decline will continue to be rapid." She pauses, taking in David's reaction. "It looks to me like her systems are shutting down." Again, she pauses. These are big words.

"Helen tells me that she is ready to come to hospice to die. We do have a bed, but I have to phone our physician to make sure that we can have it."

David is completely still for a few moments. Joanne and I say nothing. Finally, he nods his head in silent agreement. As he lowers his face, he swipes the tears that have begun to fall. His face still lowered, he manages to ask, "How long does she have?"

"Helen, is that a question that you would like to know too?" I ask. She nods. I look to Joanne, even though I have an idea myself.

Joanne says, "Helen, do you have a sense of how long you might have?" There is a long pause, and Helen whispers, "Not long."

"Is that what you are thinking too David?" He nods.

"I think that you are right, we are probably looking at short days, maybe a bit more ... but maybe not." She pauses to give them time to take this in. Knowing something inside and saying it out loud are two different things.

"How is it for you to hear those words spoken, Helen?" I ask.

"I'm at peace," she says quietly.

"And you, David?"

David rises from the couch and tentatively moves over to the bed. Like his daughter Andrea, he lays his cheek on Helen's. My eyes begin to sting, and I turn away.

After a moment, Joanne says, "I'd like to call the doctor, and if she agrees, I'll call for transport. Do you mind if I go into the kitchen?"

"No, go ahead," murmurs David.

I catch her eye and implore her to wait a minute.

"If the ambulance comes within the next hour Helen, will that be okay with you?" I ask.

Both Helen and David nod.

"I'd like to go and talk to the girls?" I look questioningly towards David.

He stares at me blankly, as if he cannot comprehend my words. I wait, suspended in motion, but he nods his head.

"I'd like to see if they have any questions, and I'll fill them in on what's happening, if that's okay with you," I say softly.

I walk through the kitchen and out onto the patio, where Cathy is playing with an electronic toy and Andrea is jumping on a small trampoline at the back of the property.

I take a seat at the table, and Cathy puts her device down, looking questioningly at me. Although I have worked with children, I'm not as comfortable with them as I am with adults. I take a deep breath, not sure of what I am going to say.

"Well, Cathy," I begin, "I've just been talking with your grandmother and your dad ..."

Her head drops.

"What have you been told so far?"

"That grandma is very, very sick."

"That's right," I say. I wait a minute.

"Is she going to die?" she blurts out.

"Yes, Cathy, I'm sorry to say that she is. No one knows for sure when that will be, but we are seeing some signs that tell us that her body is not working properly, and that it is not going to get better. She can't eat or drink anymore, and she can't get out of bed, either."

She takes a moment before asking, "Is she scared?"

"She doesn't seem to be, but you can ask her yourself," I say, trying to be as gentle as possible. She gives me a wide-eyed look, which prompts me to say, "Sometimes people can feel a bit scared when someone they love is dying."

She nods.

"Are you feeling scared?"

"Yes." Her voice is barely audible.

"It can help if you know what is going to happen. Maybe you'd like me to tell you?"

"Yes," she says firmly.

"We are going to take her to hospice, which is like a hospital, but it's a special place where people are cared for when they are dying," I begin.

I then go on to explain that her grandma will be kept comfortable and will most likely feel very peaceful, drifting in and out of sleep. In the next few days, she will most likely be sleeping for longer and longer periods, until at some point, her breaths will have long pauses between them and then, finally, she won't take another breath. At that point, her heart will stop, too. I explain that there will be nurses and doctors who will make sure that she is completely comfortable.

"You and Andrea and your mom and dad can be at her side as long as you want," I reassure her, confident from my conversation with David that the plan is for the family to be at her side at hospice.

After a pause, Cathy looks me in the eye and states, "I want her to pass away as quickly as possible, because that's what she would want." In that moment, she seems old beyond her years. I sit quietly as she lays her head on the table and sobs.

"Why are you crying?" Andrea says, walking over, obviously alarmed. "Why is she crying?" This time the question is directed at me.

Motioning for her to sit, I ask her what she thinks is happening.

"Grandma's really sick. Is she going to die?" she asks.

I go over pretty much the same things that I just talked to Cathy about. Cathy continues to cry quietly as I speak with her sister.

Andrea looks over at Cathy and says, "It's really hard for Cathy, because she and grandma are so close."

Andrea seems quite chipper as she tells me about their trip to Hawaii. The highlight for her was going to a pineapple factory with Cathy and Helen. When she starts to talk about the plans they had for the summer, I see her chin and lower lip begin to tremble. She moves her chair closer to me, and I reach out and put my arms around her, rocking her while she cries. We sit like that for some time until she abruptly wriggles free and, her face brightening, she says, "Will I get to keep her cellphone?"

I'm not sure how to respond, but Cathy does. "This is not the time to ask that," she says sharply.

I continue to answer Andrea's questions, when once again she bursts out, "Will we get all of grandma's money, because I love money," which triggers a very fierce look from Cathy.

Feeling the need to intervene, I say, "It's kind of funny what pops into your head. It's okay to have lots of different kinds of questions."

Trying to redirect the conversation, I ask them if they would like to know what will happen next. When they agree, I tell them, "We are going to take your grandma to the hospice, where it is our job to make sure that she doesn't suffer."

Andrea's mouth falls open. Obviously alarmed, she says, "Is grandma suffering?"

'Oh-oh', I think, 'wrong choice of words'. I've introduced a thought that had never occurred to Andrea. What do I say now?

"No, I don't think that she has been suffering, but we want to do everything we can to keep it that way."

I tell them that they can expect there will be lots of tears in the next while, and that it's okay, because it's normal to cry when you love someone and they are dying.

"I can tell how much you both love your grandma," I say, "and I know that she loves you too."

We sit quietly until a pretty woman walks in and introduces herself as Jane, Helen's daughter-in-law. She is beautifully dressed, but I can see that her brow is furrowed, and she looks like she hasn't slept well for a while. She has returned from the pharmacy with Helen's medication, and after a brief conversation with the others, has joined us on the patio. It looks as if she has been crying. She asks the girls to come with her to the family room.

I go into the living room and check in with Joanne and David, finding out that the ambulance is on its way. Joanne says that they are really busy today, but that they will get here as soon as they can. I return to the patio, thinking that I might as well get started on my charting, as it could be a long wait.

When Jane and the girls return, there are more questions. After letting them know that the ambulance is on its way, I assure them that when they get to Meadowview, they can sit with their grandmother if they want to, or they can go into the lounge and watch television or listen to music if they don't want to be in the room. After a pause, Cathy asks me what a dead person looks like.

"That's a really good question," I say. I want to explain it in a way that they are able to imagine "someone," but not specifically their grandma. Choosing my words carefully, I say, "When a person dies, after they have taken their last breath, they are very still. They look pale, and their skin might look a little bit like wax. Sometimes their eyes are not completely closed, and their mouth can be open, too." I pause, trying to determine whether I have said the right amount—not so graphic that it is scary, but enough to prepare them.

"Usually, you can tell that a person's spirit or life force has left, and they look peaceful, even beautiful," I add. I can tell that they are taking it in, but they don't say anything.

After a while, I notice that I am feeling restless, or maybe uneasy. I realize that it is because I am aware that this is the family's last moments at home, and I want them to take the opportunity to be with Helen. I suggest that we go back to the living room. When they are all gathered around her, Helen seems to rally her last bit of strength to assure the girls that she is comfortable and unafraid.

"I have no worries. I'm at peace," she says.

For a while, there is general conversation about their trip to Hawaii, past summers, last Christmas ... what we sometimes call "life review." When the ambulance drives up, I follow the girls as they run outside. Sylvia, the paramedic, greets them, kneeling down beside them, throwing one arm around each of them.

"How's it going?" she asks sincerely.

"It's a sad day," states Andrea. "Grandma's dying."

"That is a sad day," sympathizes Sylvia, giving them both a squeeze.

"I'll tell you what, my buddy here, Bill," indicating the man who has just gotten out of the vehicle, "is going to go and see what's up with your grandma.

Would you like to come and have a look inside the ambulance?"

"Yes!" they both exclaim, running to crawl through the open doors at the back of the van.

Paramedics in our area are equipped with the knowledge, skills and abilities to intervene in life-threatening injuries and perform pre-hospital emergency care. They travel in pairs, one doing the driving and the other being first in command. I assume that, in this case, Sylvia is in charge. Returning to the house with Bill, we consult with Joanne. Soon, Sylvia and the girls return, Sylvia pushing the gurney. Bill and Sylvia stand aside and have a short conversation before Sylvia squats by the bed. Taking Helen's hand, she says in a comforting tone, "We're going to take you for a ride to hospice. Would you like to make any stops on the way?"

No answer. Making a good guess, she asks, "Would you like to go by the river?"

Helen's eyes dart to Sylvia, but she still doesn't make a sound.

"She's always loved the river," David interjects.

Bill and Sylvia move closer, and with calculated movements, they cautiously slide Helen onto the gurney, wrapping the blankets snuggly and very precisely around her. They have intuitively picked up that Helen is fastidious and have guessed that it would be comforting to her to have the blankets tidy.

"Now, Helen," says Sylvia "is there anything we can do to make you more comfortable?"

Helen closes her eyes, a gesture that seems to mean, 'no there is nothing more that you can do'.

"Okay then, here we go," says Bill.

They wheel her out into the sunshine and onto the driveway beside the ambulance. The family clusters with Joanne and I, near the doorway to the house, looking a bit unsure. But Sylvia returns and speaks sensitively, "I want to give each of you a chance to say goodbye. You can hug Helen. You can kiss her. You can say whatever you want or need to say to her. This is your time."

Andrea is the first to go, with the others following one by one.

Sylvia keeps interjecting reassuring words. "Take your time ... you're doing fine ... that's right."

When each of them has taken a turn, Sylvia asks them if anyone would like to come in the ambulance with Helen. David volunteers. The plan is for his wife to follow in the car with the girls. As they push the stretcher into the ambulance and David climbs in behind, Joanne and I turn back towards the house and gather our bags.

Our mood is somber as we drive back to the hospital, pulling in behind the ambulance. We know that what we have witnessed is special, but it's not until we arrive back on the unit that we really understand. After Helen has been delivered safely to her room and transferred to the bed, I see Sylvia in the hall. "How did things go?" I ask.

"It was so beautiful!" says Sylvia.

David joins us. He tearfully relates how they drove to the river and opened the doors of the ambulance, pulling the stretcher out so that Helen could see the river and feel the sun on her face one last time. I feel my eyes filling with tears and I see that Joanne is also crying. David tells us that Helen then made a request to go to Tim Horton's to get a donut. Sylvia and Bill were happy to accommodate. We all know that Helen will never eat that donut. David then looks at Sylvia and says, "I don't know what I can say that will express how grateful I am that you gave my mom the chance to go to the river. It just means so much," he chokes out. Sylvia faces David and stretches her arms out so that one hand holds each of David's shoulders. Looking into his eyes before she speaks, she says, "David, I will never forget this day."

All he can manage to reply is a gruff, "Thank you."

As I walk out to the elevators with Sylvia and Bill, I turn to them and say, "You guys were amazing! I know how busy you are, how can we thank you enough for taking the time, not just with Helen, but with the whole family?"

Sylvia stops walking and looks at me, meeting my gaze. "When I get a call like this," she says, "*time stops.*"

Joanne and I never saw this family again. We can't know how much that extra time meant to them, but I am guessing that David and his wife Jane may have felt a bit unsure about sending his mom to hospice. For them, the slow pace helped them make a shift, as they watched his mom leave their home forever. For David, that time in the ambulance, by the river, was a chance to share a precious moment with his mom, and perhaps to take a breath before arriving at hospice. For the children, they saw their parents being sad, and they felt supported. They trusted Sylvia to care for their grandmother and to be sensitive to her, as she had been with them. For Helen, she had a chance to make the transition. She must have felt special, like she really mattered, instead of feeling like a burden. For all of us, images of sirens and flashing lights were replaced with the peace and stillness that comes when the people you are with are actually present, and not in a hurry to just get the job done.

Like Sylvia, actually because of Sylvia, I too will never forget this day.

ENDINGS

Spiritual leaders talk about presence and recommend the practice of being in the moment. Focusing, on a daily basis, on being present and being kind has been more than a job and more than a mission for me. It became a spiritual practice that has allowed me to serve others, and in the process, it has helped me to grow towards becoming the kind of person I wanted to be. Although in 20 years I would expect to evolve no matter what work I did, there seems to have been a kind of transformational aspect to the work, which I hope that I have conveyed.

Elisabeth Kübler-Ross, one of the pioneers of palliative care, wrote in *Death: The Final Stage of Growth* (1975):

> There is no need to be afraid of death. It is not the end of the physical body that should worry us. Rather, our concern must be to live while we're alive—to release our inner selves from the

spiritual death that comes with living
behind a façade designed to conform
to external definitions of who and what
we are. Every individual human being
born on this earth has the capacity to
become a unique and special person
unlike any who has ever existed before
or will ever exist again. But to the extent
that we become captives of culturally
defined role expectations and behav-
iours—stereotypes, not ourselves—we
block our capacity for self-actualization.
We interfere with our becoming all that
we can be. Death is the key to the door of
life. It is through accepting the finiteness
of our individual existence that we are
enabled to find the strength and courage
to reject those extrinsic roles and expectations and to devote each day of our
lives—however long they may be—to
growing as fully as we are able. p. 64

While I would not presume to say whether or not
another person needs to feel afraid of death, or what
would happen to others were they to place themselves near death as I have done, I can say that, for
me, by being willing to be in the presence of death,
I have experienced a sense of my own opening and
closing, surrender and resistance to the flow of life.
By being able to operate within the tensions and

paradoxes that encountering mortality has provided, and by being willing to show up every day, I have changed. For me, in this context, there is a sense of being pulled into a more whole version of myself. The struggle to understand, to persist, to hold intense emotion, to not know, and to express myself has helped me to become, again, who I am.

There is satisfaction in having worked as a palliative care counsellor. It is not of course the whole story, and neither is it the end, at least not today, and for that I am grateful. I hope that my story will inspire readers to think about how environments have served to shape them, and if they have, I look forward to hearing those stories. Meanwhile, may I suggest that you pull those you love close, and lean into life.

REFERENCES

Front matter

Jalāl-Din Rumi (1997). The essential Rumi (C. Barks, J. Moyne, A.J. Arberry, & R. Nicholson, Transl.). New York, NY: Castle Books.

Beginnings

DiTullio, M., & MacDonald, D. (1999). The struggle for the soul of hospice: Stress, coping, and change among hospice workers. American Journal of Hospice & Palliative Medicine, 16(5), 641.

Papadatou, D. (2001). The grieving healthcare provider. Bereavement Care, 20(2), 8.

Jones, S.H. (2005). A self-care plan for hospice workers. American Journal of Hospice and Palliative Care, 22(2), 325.

Oxford English Dictionary. (2012). "Special." Oxford University Press. www.oed.com

Shah, I. (1993). When Death came to Baghdad. In I. Shah, Tales of the Dervishes: Teaching stories of the masters over the past thousand years. Arcana, USA: Penguin Books.

Chapter One

Arrien, A. (1993). The four-fold way: Walking the paths of the warrior, teacher, healer, and visionary (p. 23). San Francisco, CA: HarperCollins.

Camargo, P. (2005). What is it like for nurses to experience the death of their patients?

Duerk, J. (1993). Circle of stones: A woman's journey to herself (p. 39). San Diego, CA: LuraMedia.

Frommer, M. (2005). Living in liminal spaces of mortality. Psychoanalytic Dialogues, (15)4, 487.

Heidegger, M. (1996). Being and time (J. Stambaugh, Trans.) (p. 222). Albany, NY: State University Press. (Original work published 1953.)

Otto, R. (1958). The idea of the holy (Vol. 14). USA: Oxford University Press.

Oxford English Dictionary. "Palliate."

Phenomenology Online (p. 8). Retrieved from: www.phe-nomenologyonline.com/sources/textorium/camargo-pilar-what-is-it-like-for-nurses-to-experience-the-death-of-their-patients/

Rogers, C. (1957). The necessary and sufficient conditions of therapeutic personality change. Journal of Consulting Psychology, 21(2), 95–103.

Worden, J. W. (1996). Children and grief: When a parent dies (p. 482). New York, NY: Guilford Press.

Chapter Two

Kuhl, D. (2002). What dying people want. Toronto, ON: Doubleday Canada.

Sheard, Sarah. (1985). Almost Japanese. New York, NY: Charles Scribner's Sons.

Chapter Four

Breiddal, S. (2013). Dwelling in the realm of death: The lived experience of counsellors' encounters with mortality in a palliative care context (pp. 125–126). University of Victoria, Victoria BC.

Joseph, E. (2010). Intimate strangers. <u>Malahat Review</u>, <u>173</u>, <u>Winter</u>, 12.

Rokach, A. (2005). Caring for those who care for the dying: Coping with the demands of palliative care workers. <u>Palliative and Supportive Care</u>, <u>3(4)</u>, 327.

Chapter Five

Cappon, D. (1994). <u>Intuition and management: Research and application</u> (p. 22). Westport, USA: Quorom Books.

Denzin, N., & Lincoln, Y. (2005). <u>The discipline and practice of qualitative research</u> (p. 24). In E. G. Guba & Y. S. Lincoln (Eds.), <u>Sage handbook of qualitative research</u> (3rd ed.) (pp. 1–32). Thousand Oaks, CA: Sage.

Gee, J. (2000). Identity as an analytic lens for research in education. <u>Review of Research in Education</u>, <u>25(99)</u>, 99–125. Accessed at: http://journals.sagepub.com/doi/abs/10.3102/0091732X025001099

Chapter Seven

Gergen, K. (1985). The social constructionist movement in modern psychology. <u>American Psychologist</u>, <u>40(3)</u>.

Papadatou, D. (2010). Taylor and Francis.

Chapter Nine

Carse, J. (1986). <u>Finite and infinite games</u> (pp. 18–19). New York, NY: Free Press.

Rosenberg, M. (2003). <u>Nonviolent communication: A language of life</u>. Encinitas, CA: PuddleDancer Press.

Chapter Ten

Groom, C., & Pennebaker, J. (2002). Words. <u>Journal of Research in Personality, 36(6)</u>, 615–621.

Endings

Kübler-Ross, E. (1975). <u>Death: The final stage of growth</u> (p. 64). New York, NY: Prentice-Hall.

ACKNOWLEDGEMENTS

I would like to thank my colleagues, family and friends who read this manuscript and gave me extensive feedback. Without their effusive encouragement, I would not have continued.

Thank you to Lisa Leighton for understanding what I was trying to do, and for taking on the editing of this book.

I would also like to express my love for my family of origin: my parents Jane and Bill Fownes, and my siblings, Diane, Karen, David and Lynda, and ask for their forgiveness for the things that I have said or not said, and done and not done, that may have hurt them. For these, I am deeply sorry. You have stayed the journey with me and I am so grateful for your presence.

About the Author

Susan Breiddal, PhD, lives in Victoria with her husband of 45 years, Bruce. She is a person of whole-hearted passion, whether tackling mothering, palliative care, rock climbing, cooking and entertaining, Duplicate Bridge, CrossFit, or eating candy. She has, however, been known to neglect parts of her life that do not interest her (housework, politics, tofu, and finances). Being kind, connecting with those she loves, practicing gratitude, and having fun are her main areas of interest these days.

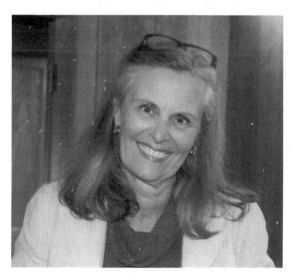